ULTRASOUND OF MOUSE FETAL DEVELOPMENT AND HUMAN CORRELATES

ULTRASOUND OF MOUSE FETAL DEVELOPMENT AND HUMAN CORRELATES

Mary C. Peavey MD, MSCI
Assistant Professor, Department of Obstetrics and Gynecology, Director,
UNC Fertility Preservation Program, Reproductive Endocrinology and
Infertility, University of North Carolina, Chapel Hill, NC, USA

and

Sarah K. Dotters-Katz MD
Assistant Professor, Department of Obstetrics and Gynecology, Duke
University School of Medicine, Durham, NC, USA

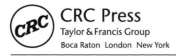

CRC Press
Taylor & Francis Group
Boca Raton London New York

CRC Press is an imprint of the
Taylor & Francis Group, an **informa** business

First edition published 2021
by CRC Press
6000 Broken Sound Parkway NW, Suite 300, Boca Raton, FL 33487-2742

and by CRC Press
2 Park Square, Milton Park, Abingdon, Oxon, OX14 4RN

© 2021 Taylor & Francis Group, LLC

CRC Press is an imprint of Taylor & Francis Group, LLC

Library of Congress Cataloging-in-Publication Data
Names: Peavey, Mary C., author. | Dotters-Katz, Sarah K., author.
Title: Ultrasound of mouse fetal development and human correlates / Mary C. Peavey, Sarah K. Dotters-Katz.
Description: First edition. | Boca Raton : CRC Press, 2021. | Series: Reproductive medicine and assisted reproductive techniques series | Includes bibliographical references and index.
Identifiers: LCCN 2020049417 (print) | LCCN 2020049418 (ebook) | ISBN 9781138071247 (hardback) | ISBN 9781138071216 (paperback) | ISBN 9781315114736 (ebook)
Subjects: LCSH: Mice--Embryology--Laboratory manuals. | Mice--Development--Laboratory manuals. | Fetus--Development--Laboratory manuals. | Mice as laboratory animals. | Animal models in research.
Classification: LCC QL737.R666 P43 2021 (print) | LCC QL737.R666 (ebook) | DDC 616.02/7333--dc23
LC record available at https://lccn.loc.gov/2020049417
LC ebook record available at https://lccn.loc.gov/2020049418q

ISBN: 978-1-138-07124-7 (hbk)
ISBN: 978-1-138-07121-6 (pbk)
ISBN: 978-1-315-11473-6 (ebk)

Typeset in Times
by MPS Limited, Dehradun

Contents

Acknowledgements..vi

Foreword by Carlos Simon and Cecilia Valdes...vii

Preface...ix

Chapter 1 Implantation and Embryonic Imaging: Mouse until D4.5–9.5;
Human 5–9 Weeks 1

Chapter 2 Early Organogenesis and First Trimester: Mouse D10.5–12.5;
Human 9–12 Weeks 15

Chapter 3 Mid-Gestation and Second Trimester: Mouse D13.5–15.5;
Human 13–27 Weeks 31

Chapter 4 Central Nervous System and Facial Development:
Mouse D13.5–15.5; Human 13–27 Weeks...45

Chapter 5 Late-Gestation and Third Trimester: Mouse D16.5–18.5;
Human 28–40 Weeks 59

Chapter 6 Placenta Throughout Gestation 75

Index...87

Acknowledgements

The completion of this work would not be possible without the incredible support from many mentors and colleagues. I am grateful to Dr. William Gibbons, a beacon in the field of reproductive biology, for his clinical guidance and wisdom to expand this translational research. I would especially like to thank scientific mentors Dr. Franco DeMayo and Dr. John Lydon, who served as resources for murine research, encouraged the growth of this fetal ultrasound technique, and offered the resources to push the boundaries of prenatal ultrasonography in mice. Additionally, as special recognition to Dr. Carlos Simon for his support and encouragement in the development and publication of this work.

I have extraordinary appreciation for Dr. Corey Reynolds who provided the technical assistance for specialized mouse ultrasonography. I also offer a special recognition of Dr. Cecilia Valdes, Dr. Amy Schutt, and Dr. Neil Chappell for serving as outstanding role models for physician scientists.

A most special thank you to my husband, Dr. Daniel Landi, for supporting this book from cover to cover.

Foreword

Human pregnancy is one of the most fascinating and enigmatic events for humankind, but also a key indicator of the overall health of a community, country, or continent. Given that perinatal mortality accounts for two-thirds of infant deaths, it is understandable why optimizing the content, access, and delivery of prenatal care became the major focus of obstetrics during the 20th century.

Every year, an estimated 3.6 million infants worldwide die within the first four weeks of life. Of these, preterm labor and delivery (which affect 10% of all births), and preeclampsia (5%) contribute to 1.5 million neonatal deaths during the first week of life and to 1.4 million stillborn babies. Congenital anomalies affect 2–3% of newborns whose parents conceived naturally. Genetic disorders affect 1% of live births and are responsible for 18% of pediatric hospitalizations and 20% of infant mortality. Many of these genetic disorders are caused by recessive or X-linked genetic mutations carried by 85% of humans.

Physicians have been trying to assess the course of pregnancy from the most remote antiquity. Before ultrasound, obstetrics had little more to offer gravid women than tender, loving care hoping for a normal baby. Maternal Fetal Medicine specialists can now visualize the course of pregnancy through different technologies enabling early, accurate diagnosis and treatment in-utero of some fetal pathologies.

Comparative research during pregnancy across species has become rare in recent years. Studies contrasting imaging throughout the different trimesters of human pregnancy versus the equivalent timing in animal models are needed. In particular comparison between human and rodent pregnancy is interesting given the many research and translational possibilities. This is precisely the topic of this interesting book, a systematic visual comparison to identify common mechanisms underlying obstetrical pathologies and fetal abnormalities in murine and human pregnancy.

This knowledge is of interest to clinicians and researchers in preconception and prenatal care. Prenatally, the complexities of pregnancy necessitate continued basic and clinical research, since malformations and/or malfunctions lead to compromised pregnancy outcomes and may even impact the long-term health of offspring that can be assessed only with short-lifespan mammals. Pre-conception care aims to optimize gestational outcome before pregnancy is established. Multiple lines of evidence have now coalesced to support the concept that most complications of pregnancy emerge from disorders which have their origins in early pregnancy, at the time of implantation and placentation. An accumulating body of knowledge indicates that environmental factors have a profound effect on lifetime health (e.g., diet, body composition, metabolism, and stress). This is now so compelling that it calls for revisiting and reframing the advice provided to parents preparing for pregnancy. This volume offers a great opportunity for human ART researchers in the understanding and study of these variables that affect the in utero environment.

Dr. Mary Peavey is a true physician scientist. She developed the techniques illustrated in this extraordinary book while training as a fellow at Baylor College of Medicine (BCM)/Texas Children's Hospital Pavilion for Women in Reproductive Endocrinology and Infertility. Can you imagine developing and then performing detailed, individual obstetrical ultrasounds on fetuses the size of a grain of rice in a uterus containing eight fetuses? "Translational research" is the goal of research training for MDs with clinical knowledge to inform basic science to achieve "bench to bedside" applications of research. Dr. Peavey's translational skills are bi-directional: she brought her obstetrical ultrasound skills with humans to her mouse research subjects resulting in a less invasive, more ethical and more efficient method to study ongoing mouse pregnancy, and she has been able to guide her basic mouse research in progesterone receptor isoforms to improve understanding of human pregnancy and the onset of labor. She is an example of the value of programs such as the NIH designed Clinical Scientist Training Program, in which she trained while at BCM, and that strive to promote such essential and applicable research. It is an honor to have watched Dr. Peavey develop and now share her knowledge.

Dr. Sarah Dotters-Katz is the epitome of a physician educator and researcher, with a career dedicated to the growth and development of junior physicians while actively contributing to the field of maternal and fetal medicine. After completing her general Obstetrics and Gynecology Residency at Duke University Medical Center with co-author Dr. Peavey, Dr. Dotters-Katz subsequently received her subspecialty training in Maternal and Fetal Medicine at the University of North Carolina. As the early mouse imaging of the comparative anatomy was developed, Dr. Dotters-Katz joined the project, using her skills in human fetal ultrasound to provide appropriate human correlates to the mouse ultrasounds. As one will see, she has an innate ability to capture and describe the relevant fetal anatomy that bridges both mice and humans alike. Her success as a clinician educator derives from her intrinsic skills to synthesize complex information and present it in a concise manner for learners. This, in combination with her continued training via a Masters Medical Health Professions Education and her specialist training in ultrasound and fetal anatomy, has provided this publication with a unique yet approachable view of how humans and mice are more alike during development than we would first assume.

The chapters in this book cover advances in the comparative imaging of human and mouse pregnancy through different time frames (weeks vs. days post coitum [dpc]) and developing organ systems as well as the placenta. Many of the comparative imaging concepts should serve to both inform and inspire readers, clinicians, researchers, and embryologists to continue pushing the boundaries of knowledge of the enigmas of human pregnancy.

Carlos Simon
Department of Obstetrics & Gynecology, School of Medicine
Valencia University Igenomix Foundation, INCLIVA, Spain
Department of Obstetrics and Gynecology, BIDMC Harvard University
Boston, Massachusetts, USA
Department of Obstetrics & Gynecology, Baylor College of Medicine
Houston, Texas, USA

Cecilia Valdes
Department of Obstetrics & Gynecology, Baylor College of Medicine
Houston, Texas, USA

Preface

As is often the case with the development of new techniques, the comparative images of murine and human fetal anatomy were a product of both necessity and opportunity. While exploring the options for phenotyping abnormal pregnancy outcomes in our own mouse model, we decided to use the most common tool used as obstetricians — the ultrasound. Even from the onset, the obvious similarities of mouse and fetal anatomy via ultrasound were striking. The convergence of our subspecialty medical training in obstetrical human ultrasounds and prior work in characterizing mouse pregnancies provided the opportunity to use human-based ultrasound technique in the 'mouse obstetrical' world. What became a tool for us to answer our own investigational questions grew into an inclusive comparative atlas to be used in a large spectrum of translational research.

Studying human pathology via animal models has long been used to understand and treat human disease. However, diseases that affect human fetal development and pregnancy are especially difficult to investigate in people, due to both logistical and ethical concerns. Therefore, the increasing sophistication and use of mouse models in reproduction — particularly in maternal and fetal health during pregnancy — have great utility. The use of ultrasound in human maternal and fetal medicine, through the development of the field of obstetrics and gynecology, has improved the health and millions of mothers and babies. While the use of ultrasonography during human obstetrical care has been widely used and continues to grow in complexity, there is unfortunately a lack of comparative ultrasonography for those interested in mouse fetal development. This limits the capability of reproductive mouse models to investigate human disease.

In consideration of this, we aim to deliver a comprehensive visual comparison of mouse and human fetal anatomy to assist a variety of audiences. This text will provide basic science researchers both the technique of fetal ultrasonography and understanding of the possibilities of monitoring their specific mouse models in real-time. This avoids the alternative of having to euthanize, dissect or use histological sectioning to evaluate the anatomy, development and viability of fetuses during gestation. In addition, these ultrasound techniques promote the principles of performing more humane animal research via a reduction in animal use per experiment, as the same mice can provide numerous time points during pregnancy without termination of pregnancy, and refinement, as this non-invasive ultrasound modification minimizes pain and discomfort. Additionally, this text will give the clinician scientists the ability to understand how mouse models of human maternal and fetal disease can be surveilled and modeled in a mouse model.

In summary, this text provides the bridge between basic animal science and human maternal-fetal pathology to improve current animal model use and promote innovative new modeling of disease. We are optimistic that clinicians and scientists can utilize this text to promote the growing field of reproductive medicine.

Mary Peavey, MD, MSCI
Assistant Professor, Department of Ob-Gyn
Division of Reproductive Endocrinology and Infertility
University of North Carolina
Chapel Hill, North Carolina, USA

Sarah Dotters-Katz, MD, MMHPE
Assistant Professor, Department of Obstetrics and Gynecology
Division of Maternal Fetal Medicine
Duke University Medical Center
Durham, North Carolina, USA

1 Implantation and Embryonic Imaging
Mouse until D4.5–9.5; Human 5–9 Weeks

DATING

In the human, the first trimester marks the development of a zygote into a recognizable human fetus and is most commonly dated in relation to the first day of the last menstrual period of the mother. Consequently, the traditional dating of a human pregnancy is 2 weeks more than the actual embryological development of the pregnancy. In the mouse pregnancy, a vaginal plug is seen on the morning after copulation, and traditionally, the pregnancy is dated as this morning as being day 0.5 of pregnancy, or 0.5 days post coitus (dpc). Subsequent description of gestational dating in the human and mouse will thus be assigned as per this nomenclature.

IMAGING

In humans, during the first trimester of pregnancy, transvaginal approach provides the most accurate and reliable images of the pregnancy. In the mouse, transvaginal ultrasonography technology has yet to be developed; however the images obtained by the transabdominal approach are currently more than adequate for early gestation imaging; all mouse images were obtained with the use of the Vevo 2100 system from Fujifilm VisualSonics, as previously published (1,2). In both human and murine pregnancies, early ultrasound allows for detection of the number and location of intrauterine pregnancies, assign a gestational age and developmental of the pregnancy, and to evaluate the whether there are sonographic findings indicative of early pregnancy compromise or failure.

PREIMPLANTATION DEVELOPMENT

Similarly to human ovulation and fertilization, the mouse embryo after ovulation is transported through the fallopian tube, where fertilization with sperm occurs. The fertilized oocyte is known as the zygote, which will continue to divide into an embryo. As the embryo travels through the fallopian tube, it continues to undergo cell division; by the third day, the embryo is approximately eight cells and begins compaction. On its fifth day of growth, the human embryo has developed into a blastocyst and travels to the uterus where it begins the process of implantation and further growth. At this point, as in humans, the blastocyst consists of a discrete inner cell mass, within a spherical cavity lined by the trophectoderm cell layer. These preimplantation events cannot be ascertained via ultrasonographic methods in either the human or mouse. However, the non pregnant uterus, consisting of the myometrium and endometrium can be easily measured via sonographic methods. See Fig. 1.1.

(a)   (b)

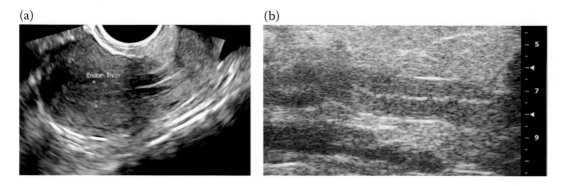

FIGURE 1.1   **A:** The non-pregnant human uterus, with trilaminar endometrial lining pattern. **B:** The non pregnant mouse uterus during proestrus, appearing as an echogenic linear line in the middle of the longitudinal uterine horn.

DECIDUALIZATION AND EARLY IMPLANTATION

Changes within the endometrium in early pregnancy can be easily identified by ultrasonography, in which the endometrium appears increased in echogenicity and thickness, in both the human as well as the mouse (3–5). The decidualized endometrium is the functional layer of the edematous and thickened endometrium in which successful implantation must occur (6,7). This change in the endometrium, prior to the development of a gestational sac correlate to 4–5 weeks gestational age in humans and 3.5–6.5 dpc in the mouse.

HUMAN

The blastocyst consists of a discrete inner cell mass, within a spherical cavity lined by the trophectoderm cell layer. In humans, by the end of the third gestational week, the blastocyst begins to implant into the decidualized endometrium. In successful pregnancies, the average endometrial thickness is 17 ± 6.7 mm (8), and the distinct echogenic decidualized endometrium can be easily identified on transvaginal ultrasound, before the presence of a gestational sac. The endometrium will continue to appear thickened and echogenic from 4 to 5 weeks gestation, before the gestational sac is visible.

MOUSE

In the mouse by 3.5 dpc, the endometrium itself remains linear in appearance without discrete sites of implantation detectable; the hyperechoic endometrium is approximately 0.14–0.2 mm in thickness. However, by 4.5 dpc, the discrete locations of embryo implantation sites can be identified, as represented by a small hyperechoic dot in the middle of the expanding myometrium. By 5.5 dpc, these discrete implantation sites are easily identified and counted, allowing for the number of implantation sites as well as the spacing interval, to be determined. The average distance between each implantation site be quantified. In this animal model, at 5.5 dpc, the average normal distance between implantation sites has been determined to be 1.8–2 mm (2). At 6.5 dpc, the uterus begins to take on a distinct spherical shape around each implantation site, causing each uterine horn to resemble "a string of pearls" on ultrasound imaging. The bright areas of decidualized endometrium continue to reveal distinct endometrial implantation sites are easily identifiable; at this stage, the average spacing between each implantation site is 2.99 ± 0.3 mm (2). See Figs. 1.2–1.5.

(a)

(b)

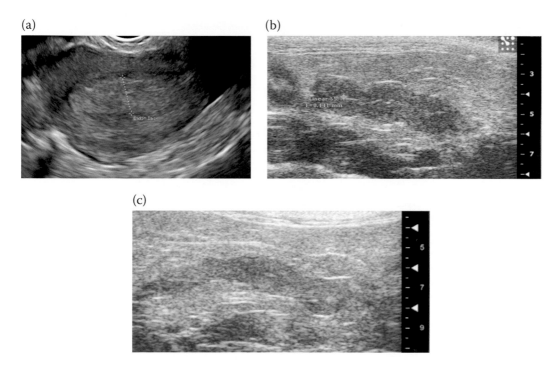

(c)

FIGURE 1.2 **A:** The human endometrium during very early pregnancy, which is thickened at a gestational age of 4 weeks and 3 days. **B:** The mouse pregnancy at 3.5 dpc, with the slight appearance of three rounded implantation sites in the longitudinal uterine horn. **C:** The same mouse pregnancy at 4.5 dpc, with the bright echogenic implantation sites now easily visible and loss of echogenicity between implantation sites.

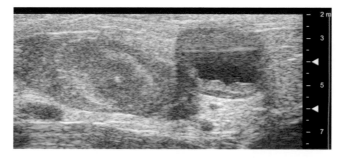

FIGURE 1.3 The early pregnant mouse pregnancy, seen here at 4.5 dpc, with a bright, echogenic sphere in the center of the expanding uterine horn. The maternal bladder is seen to the right.

(a)   (b)

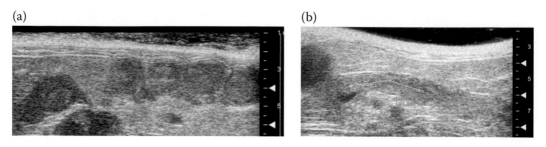

FIGURE 1.4   A: The mouse pregnancy at 5.5 dpc, with four implantation sites seen in the right horn and the most proximal implantation site on the left horn. **B:** The mouse pregnancy at 5.5 dpc, with the distance between implantation sites measurable.

(a)   (b)

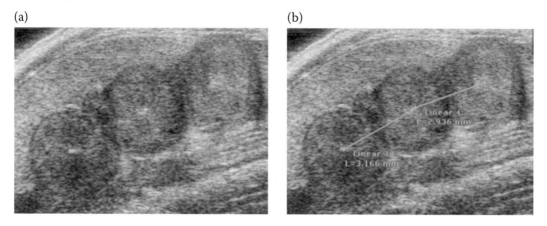

FIGURE 1.5   A: The mouse pregnancy at 6.5 dpc; three implantation sites are now easily visualized as distinct sites, within one uterine horn. **B:** The mouse pregnancy at 6.5 dpc; the distance between each implantation site is easily quantified, as shown measured.

DEVELOPMENT OF GESTATIONAL SAC

The first reliable sonographic evidence of an early intrauterine pregnancy in both the human and mouse is the presence of a gestational sac (9,10). A gestational sac is identified as a small, round, anechoic fluid collection surrounded by the hyperechoic rim of endometrial tissue. In both mice and in humans the mean sac diameter (MSD) can be obtained by measuring the diameter of the sac in each of three dimensions and then averaging the measurements (11). The gestational sac, is first visible at the fifth week of gestation in the human and at 7.5 dpc in the mouse pregnancy.

HUMAN

In humans, the position of the gestational sac should be in the mid to upper uterus. The shape should be round and fairly spherical in its dimensions. In humans, as early as the fifth week of pregnancy, a yolk sac within the gestational sac is the first sonographic confirmation of a developing intrauterine pregnancy. A pseudogestational sac can sometimes be seen in the instance of an ectopic or extra-uterine pregnancy, but would not contain a yolk sac.

MOUSE

In the mouse, a gestational sac should form at each implantation site, which should remain roughly equally distributed throughout each horn, both proximally and distally. Similar to human development, the gestational sac is visualized as a small, round, anechoic area in the site of the implantation area. The appearance of a gestational sac reliably occurs between 6.5 and 7.5 dpc. The absence of a gestational sac on 7.5 dpc confirms an abnormal pregnancy that will not progress into a viable pregnancy. See Figs. 1.6 and 1.7.

(a)   (b)

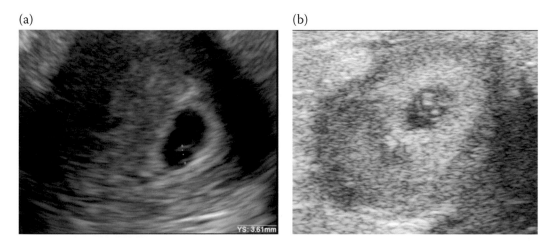

FIGURE 1.6   A: A human pregnancy 5 weeks and 3 days, with a normal appearing yolk sac within the gestational sac. **B:** A mouse pregnancy 7.5 dpc, with a gestational sac and likely the beginning growth of the fetus. In this instance, the measurements of the gestational sac are 1.1 × 0.7 × 0.8 mm, with a mean sac diameter (MSD) of 0.87 mm. A small echogenic area, likely a small fetal pole, is measured at 0.5 mm.

(a)   (b)

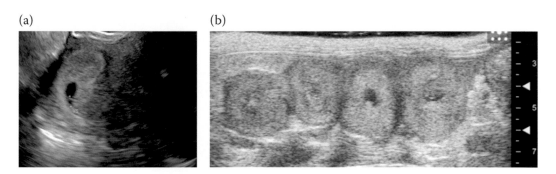

FIGURE 1.7   A: A human pregnancy 5 weeks and 6 days; with a normal appearing yolk sac within the gestational sac. **B:** A mouse pregnancy on 7.5 dpc, with four gestational sacs in one uterine horn (note: not all sacs were visible in the same plane).

DETECTION OF A FETAL POLE

The first signs of fetal development and growth is the detection of a fetal pole, an elongated oval-shaped hyperechoic structure within the anechoic gestational sac. In humans, the fetal pole can first be detected between 6 and 7 weeks gestation, while in the mouse the fetal pole is first detected between 7.5 and 8.5 dpc. Measurements of a fetal pole are described as the crown rump length (CRL), which measures the distance between the two ends of the most elongated view of the fetal pole. Discrete fetal structures and polarity cannot be detected in this very early developmental stage.

Human

In humans, a fetal crown rump length (CRL) can be detected as early as 6 weeks gestation, and reliably by 7 weeks gestation. If the mean sac diameter is ≥25 mm and no embryo is identified, this is concerning for an abnormal, non-viable pregnancy (12), while a mean sac diameter of 16–24 mm without an embryo raises suspicion for, but it not diagnostic of, a failed pregnancy (12).

Mouse

While a hint of a developing fetus may be seen in some implantation sites on the evening of 7.5 dpc, the murine fetal pole will reliably be visualized at 8.5 dpc in all viable pregnancy sites. The development of the mouse fetus is rapid between 7.5 and 9.5 dpc, and differences in fetal measurements can be appreciated between early morning and late afternoon ultrasounds on the same day. The absence of a fetal pole or a measurable CRL at 8.5 dpc confirms an abnormal pregnancy that will not continue to a viable pregnancy. See Fig. 1.8.

(a)   (b)

(c)

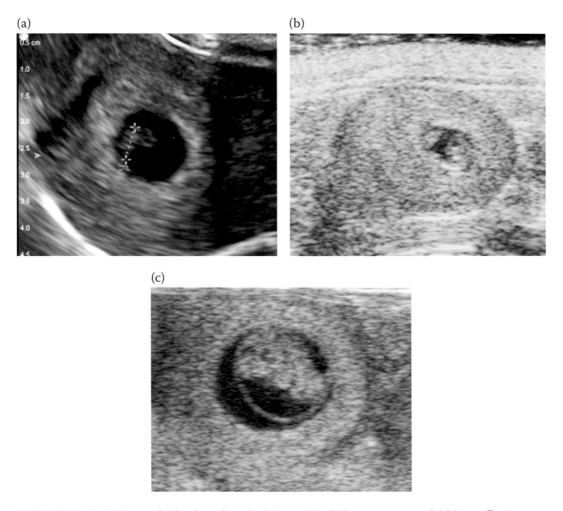

FIGURE 1.8   A: A human fetal pole at 6 weeks 3 days, with CRL measurement of 6.34 mm. **B:** A mouse fetal pole within gestational sac, seen very early on the morning of 8.5 dpc and with a CRL 0.78 mm. **C:** A mouse fetal pole on the evening of 8.5 dpc, with a CRL measurement of 1.8 mm. The amnion can be first visible at this gestational age.

FETAL POLARITY AND DEVELOPMENT OF BASIC STRUCTURES

As the fetus continues to grow and develop, discrete structures indicating the fetal polarity and generation of the central nervous system and limb buds are often detectable at an early stage in both human and mouse pregnancies. The first structures are visible between 8 and 9 weeks in the human and between 8.5 and 9.5 dpc in the mouse.

HUMAN

The development of discrete structures such as fore-limb and hind-limb buds and early central nervous system are first detectable in the human fetus between 8 and 9 weeks gestation, allowing for the polarity of the growing fetus to be determined. The unfused amnion can often be detected via transvaginal ultrasound during this time frame.

MOUSE

Between days 8.5 and 9.5 dpc, the mouse fetus undergoes significant development and growth on sonographic imaging. While fore-limb and hind-limb buds begins to develop at 9.5 dpc, this is often not reliably appreciable via ultrasound on 9.5 dpc. The unfused amniotic membrane may be visible. Polarity of the fetus is visible with the fetal CNS and cephalad structures seen. By 8.5 dpc the mouse embryo initiates neural tube closure and a crown-rump length of the fetal pole is reliably measurable (1,2,13). In mice, the amnion is first visible at D8.5, and remains visible and un-fused via sonographic findings until 13.5–14.5 dpc. See Fig. 1.9.

ESTABLISHMENT, DETECTION AND QUANTIFICATION OF CARDIAC ACTIVITY

The establishment and function of the circulatory system confirms normal development and continuing reassurance of the viability of the fetus. Doppler ultrasound detection of fetal cardiac motion, as well as Doppler detection of umbilical cord blood flow can be used to document and confirm continued fetal circulation in human and mouse pregnancies.

HUMAN

The primordial heart starts to beat at 6 weeks, and rapid fetal growth and organogenesis occurs from weeks 6–10. Transvaginal ultrasonography can detect fetal cardiac activity as early as 34 gestational days, or as early as a CRL length of 1.6 mm. Cardiac activity should be routinely detected when the human embryo has reached 4–5 mm in length. The absence of a heart beat when the CRL is >4 mm confirms a non-viable fetus (12). Findings suspicious for, but not diagnostic of pregnancy failure, CRL of <7 mm and no heartbeat. In humans, the crown rump length at 10 weeks is approximately 30 mm. In humans, the amnion is not visible until at least CRL of 7 mm, or approximately 7 weeks gestational age.

MOUSE

In the mouse, cardiac activity can be detected as early as 8.5 dpc, (correlating to a CRL of 1.5 to 2 mm) although this is variable on the position of uterus and each fetus during sonographic examination. In the mouse at 9.5 dpc, the fetal circulation has developed to where both cardiac and umbilical blood flow are easily visualized sonographically. Thus the absence of detectable cardiac

(a)   (b)

(c)   (d)

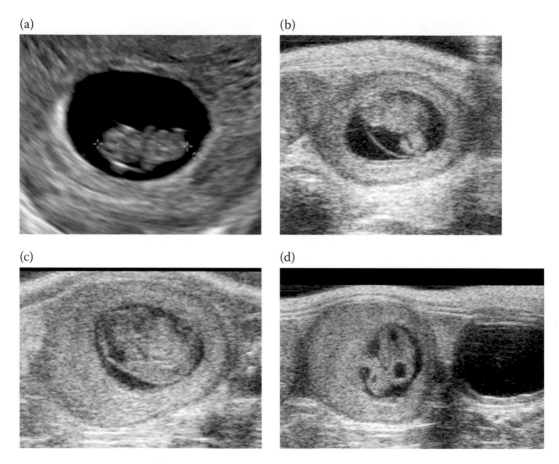

FIGURE 1.9 **A:** Human pregnancy at 8 weeks and 2 days, with a viable fetus and CRL of 21.25 mm. The cephalic and caudal regions, limb buds and cardiac activity of the fetus are easily identified. **B:** The mouse fetus at 9.5 dpc, with a CRL of 3.2 mm. The unfused amnion and umbilical cord easily visualized. **C:** Mouse fetal development at 9.5 dpc, with a CRL measuring 3.8 mm. The cephalad and caudal regions are clearly visible. **D:** Mouse fetal development at 9.5, with a CRL of 3.4 mm. This pregnancy site is the closes to the cervix in this uterine horn and the maternal bladder with urine is easily visualized at the right of the image as an anechoic structure.

activity at 9.5 dpc is conclusive of a non-viable fetus. The umbilical cord with blood flow, indicates the site of the developing placenta, and can be detected and monitored. In a mouse pregnancy which has unclear or uncertain dating, an expected CRL at 9.5 dpc (2.0–2.5 mm) is a helpful marker. Thus, in a pregnancy of unknown gestational dating, when any CRL measures >2.0 mm and no cardiac activity is seen, this is concerning for fetal demise. The absence of cardiac activity with a CRL of >2.5 mm would confirm a non-viable fetus.

FETAL HEART RATE

In both human and mouse cardiac development, the earliest detectable heart rates in beats per minute (bpm) are often lower at the time of first detection (100–120 bpm in humans and 120–150 bpm in mice). The heart rate increases rapidly during development, increasing to 140–170 bpm in humans and 200–240 bpm in mice throughout gestation. See Fig. 1.10.

(a)   (b)

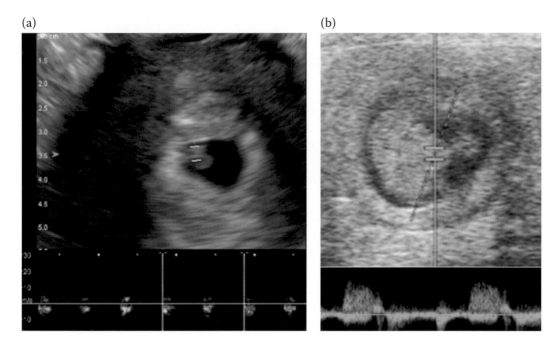

FIGURE 1.10 A: Human fetal cardiac activity is detected at 6 weeks and 1 day, at 115 bpm. The heart rate will increase over the next several weeks gestation, to levels in 160–170 bpm by 8–9 weeks gestation. **B:** Mouse fetal cardiac activity at 9.5 dpc, 117 bpm. As in humans, the cardiac rate increases, and by 10.5 dpc, is detected via umbilical cord Doppler at approximately 160 bpm.

FIRST TRIMESTER COMPLICATIONS

First trimester complications such as implantation failure, anembryonic pregnancy, and miscarriage are, unfortunately, seen commonly in clinical practice. As mouse models have been developed to study mammalian pregnancies and therapeutic interventions, the need for early pregnancy detection and assessment via ultrasound is paramount. Both abnormal human and mouse early pregnancy examples are included, for correlation, as below.

EARLY PREGNANCY LOSS

The failure of a pregnancy can occur even before the detection and development of a gestational sac. This is often seen as a thickened decidualized endometrium without an anechoic region which would indicate the presence of a gestational sac. In humans, a gestational sac should be visible as early as 5 weeks gestation, while in mice, a gestational sac should be visible at 7.5 dpc. The absence of a gestational sac at these time points is indicative of an abnormal or failed pregnancy. Previously, in the mouse, failed early pregnancies in mice have only been described via dissection, after the animal has already been euthanized. By dissection, a failed early pregnancy is seen as a small, darker pinpoint area embedded in the endometrium without a defined embryo identified. While human early pregnancy loss can be detected very early via serum human chorionic gonadotropin (hCG) levels, no such testing exists in mice. Thus, non-invasive ultrasound monitoring can provide this information without interrupting pregnancy.

ANEMBRYONIC PREGNANCY (BLIGHTED OVUM)

An anembryonic pregnancy is one in which the developmental arrest occurred either before the formation of the embryo or before ultrasonography can reliably detect fetal development. This

(a)   (b)

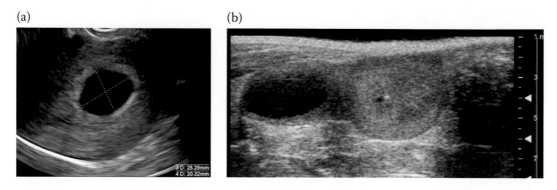

FIGURE 1.11   A: A human anembryonic pregnancy at 7 weeks and 1 day, with the presence of a large gestational sac, without a yolk sac or fetal pole visible at a mean sac diameter of 24 mm. **B:** A mouse anembryonic pregnancy at 8.5 dpc, with a small gestational sac and no fetal pole, confirming the diagnosis of anembryonic pregnancy.

results in the appearance of the gestational sac but without a fetal pole. In humans, findings diagnostic of pregnancy failure include a mean sac diameter of ≥25 mm and no embryo (12). Findings suspicious for, but not diagnostic of, pregnancy failure, mean sac diameter of 16–24 mm and no embryo (12). In mice, a mean sac diameter of >2 mm and no fetal pole is diagnostic of an anembryonic pregnancy. See Fig. 1.11.

FIRST TRIMESTER SPONTANEOUS ABORTION

In humans, useful ultrasound findings such as fetal bradycardia, intrauterine hematoma (9), lagging crown rump length and yolk sac have yielded predictive value of a pending miscarriage (4). In multifetal gestations, a significant association was found between the increase in the degree of embryonic discordance and the likelihood of early fetal loss (14).

However, prior to the development of early mouse ultrasound, no such correlation as previously existed no such correlated has previously existed for murine early pregnancy monitoring. As well-characterized in early human pregnancies, early mouse fetal ultrasound can now detect which murine pregnancies are continuing in a normal fashion, and which are at a high likelihood of failure. The described mouse modeling techniques with ultrasound allow for murine models of recurrent pregnancy loss to be documented and detected at these very early time points that are critical in early pregnancy establishment. A timeline of normal and abnormal pregnancy from 8.5 to 13.5 dpc is illustrated in the fetal growth curves as below. See Fig. 1.12.

DEVELOPMENT OF EARLY MURINE FETAL GROWTH CURVE

In early mouse pregnancy, the growth and development of each gestational site can be tracked via ultrasonography. Due to the very small size of the early decidualized endometrium and gestational sac, the measurement of each pregnancy site is more reliably calculated by the volume of the implantation site, as calculated by either 3-D ultrasound technology (1), or by approximation with three measurements in using 2-D real time ultrasonography using measurements of width, length, and height, as shown on 11.5 dpc. See Fig. 1.13.

(a)   (b)

(c)   (d)

(e)   (f)

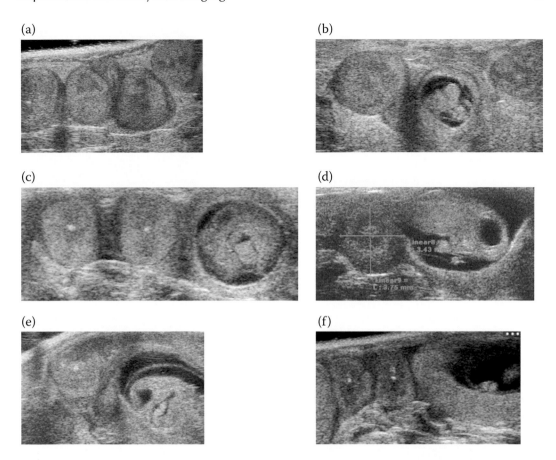

FIGURE 1.12 Mouse failed pregnancies (resorptions) from 8.5 to 13.5 dpc. **A:** 8.5 dpc. All pregnancy sites without a gestational sac or CRL in any of the four implantation sites. **B:** 9.5 dpc. Two resorptions are seen flanking a viable pregnancy in the center. **C:** 10.5 dpc. Two resorptions are seen on the left, with a viable continuing pregnancy on the right. **D:** 11.5 dpc. One resorption, with calipers measuring the total volume of the site. **E:** 12.5 dpc. One resorption, on the left, with the cephalad region of a neighboring viable pregnancy. **F:** 13.5 dpc. Two resorptions are seen on the left, with a viable continuing pregnancy on the right.

Abnormalities in fetal growth and fetal demise cab be surmised by ultrasound, plotting the growth versus normal developmental curves. Analogous to human fetal growth monitoring, the cessation or lagging of growth is concerning and indicative of pregnancy failure. Of note, the most consistent manner in which to measure the size of early mouse pregnancy sites is to determine the average mean diameter of the expanded myometrium, as demonstrated in Fig. 1.14.

SUMMARY

Early pregnancy events including decidualization, implantation, early fetal growth and the establishment of the circulatory system are intricate, critical events in the establishment of normal mammalian pregnancies. As the human and mouse have numerous developmental similarities during this process of early fetal development, advances in murine ultrasound imaging allow for mouse models to more efficiently provide translational information for continued research into normal and abnormal early pregnancy events.

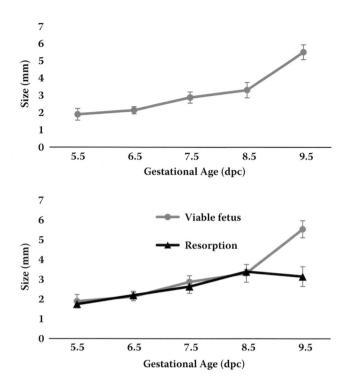

FIGURE 1.13   Early murine fetal development curve. (Graphs modified from (1,2).)

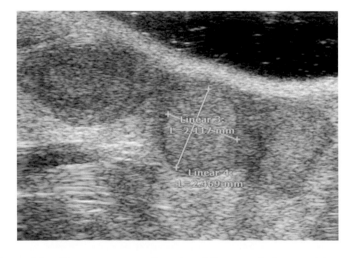

FIGURE 1.14   Determining the average mean diameter of the expanded myometrium.

REFERENCES

1. Peavey, M. C., Reynolds, C. L., Szwarc, M. M., Gibbons, W. E., Valdes, C. T., DeMayo, F. J., et al., A novel use of three-dimensional high-frequency ultrasonography for early pregnancy characterization in the mouse. *J Vis Exp*. 2017 (128): 56207. doi:10.3791/56207.
2. Peavey, M. C., Reynolds, C. L., Szwarc, M. M., Gibbons, W. E., Valdes, C. T., DeMayo, F. J., et al., Three-dimensional high-frequency ultrasonography for early detection and characterization of embryo implantation site development in the mouse. *PLoS One*. 2017. 12(1): e0169312.
3. Flores, L. E., Hildebrandt, T. B., Kuhl, A. A. and Drews, B., Early detection and staging of spontaneous embryo resorption by ultrasound biomicroscopy in murine pregnancy. *Reprod Biol Endocrinol*. 2014. 12: 38.
4. Datta, M. R. and Raut, A., Efficacy of first-trimester ultrasound parameters for prediction of early spontaneous abortion. *Int J Gynaecol Obstet*. 2017. 138(3): 325–330.
5. Yadav, P., Singla, A., Sidana, A., Suneja, A. and Vaid, N. B., Evaluation of sonographic endometrial patterns and endometrial thickness as predictors of ectopic pregnancy. *Int J Gynaecol Obstet*. 2017. 136(1): 70–75.
6. Valbuena, D., Valdes, C. T. and Simon C., Introduction: endometrial function: facts, urban legends, and an eye to the future. *Fertil Steril*. 2017. 108(1): 4–8.
7. Valdes, C. T., Schutt, A. and Simon, C., Implantation failure of endometrial origin: it is not pathology, but our failure to synchronize the developing embryo with a receptive endometrium. *Fertil Steril*. 2017. 108(1): 15–18.
8. Moschos, E. and Twickler, D. M., Endometrial thickness predicts intrauterine pregnancy in patients with pregnancy of unknown location. *Ultrasound Obstet Gynecol*. 2008. 32(7): 929–934.
9. Pillai, R. N., Konje, J. C., Richardson, M., Tincello, D. G. and Potdar, N., Prediction of miscarriage in women with viable intrauterine pregnancy – a systematic review and diagnostic accuracy meta-analysis. *Eur J Obstet Gynecol Reprod Biol*. 2018. 220: 122–131.
10. Sohaey, R., Woodward, P. and Zwiebel, W. J., First-trimester ultrasound: the essentials. *Semin Ultrasound CT MR*. 1996. 17(1): 2–14.
11. Li, X., Ouyang, Y., Yi, Y., Tan, Y. and Lu, G., Correlation analysis between ultrasound findings and abnormal karyotypes in the embryos from early pregnancy loss after in vitro fertilization-embryo transfer. *J Assist Reprod Genet*. 2017. 34(1): 43–50.
12. Doubilet, P. M., Benson, C. B., Bourne, T., Blaivas, M., Society of Radiologists in Ultrasound Multispecialty Panel on Early First Trimester Diagnosis of Miscarriage and Exclusion of a Viable Intrauterine Pregnancy, et al., Diagnostic criteria for nonviable pregnancy early in the first trimester. *N Engl J Med*. 2013. 369(15): 1443–1451.
13. Paudyal, A., Damrau, C., Patterson, V. L., Ermakov, A., Formstone, C., Lalanne, Z., et al., The novel mouse mutant, chuzhoi, has disruption of Ptk7 protein and exhibits defects in neural tube, heart and lung development and abnormal planar cell polarity in the ear. *BMC Dev Biol*. 2010. 10: 87.
14. D'Antonio, F., Khalil, A., Mantovani, E. and Thilaganathan, B., Embryonic growth discordance and early fetal loss: the STORK multiple pregnancy cohort and systematic review. *Hum Reprod*, 2013. 28(10): 2621–2627.

2 Early Organogenesis and First Trimester
Mouse D10.5–12.5; Human 9–12 Weeks

IMAGING

In humans, transabdominal ultrasound imaging becomes more useful as the first trimester ends and the second trimester begins, due to both ease of use for practitioner and patient, as well as the ability for a transabdominal ultrasound to provide a larger view of the pregnancy. In mice, a transabdominal approach still produces the most reliable images during this timeframe as well. As the fetus develops, ultrasound continues to provide the number and location of intrauterine pregnancies, fetal viability through detection of cardiac activity, monitoring of fetal growth, and development of organs.

ORGANOGENESIS

In mammalian development, each of the three germ cell layers (ectoderm, mesoderm and endoderm) undergo differentiation via intricate cellular signaling. This signaling results in further cell differentiation and organization, leading to the growth of organs. In humans, the internal organs begin to develop 3–8 weeks after fertilization. During this time, the neural system, heart, upper and lower limbs, ear, eye, palate and external genitalia are forming; any adverse exposure during this time can result in major congenital abnormalities. In mice, a majority of internal organs begin to develop between 9.5 and 11.5 dpc. Both human and mouse embryological development have been extensively characterized (1), allowing the mouse to serve as an experimental model for human disease and abnormal organogenesis.

CARDIAC

The cardiac development in mouse and human fetuses are overall quite comparable (2), with similar atrial, ventricular, and outflow septation development. Subsequently, mouse cardiac morphogenesis can be a very useful model for human development and congenital heart disease. Cardiac formation begins when the two endocardial tubes merge, forming the tubular heart (primitive heart tube), which will then loop and septate, resulting in the four-chambered heart (3).

Human

The main walls of the heart are formed between day 27 and 37 of development. With transvaginal imaging, a four-chambered heart can be identified in at least half of pregnancies in the eighth week, and increasing incrementally to 98% detection by the 11th week (4). The umbilical cord is first seen between 8 and 9 weeks gestation, at which time the umbilical cord flow is detectable via color Doppler; umbilical cord morphology can be consistently studied in the first trimester from 11 to 13 weeks (5). From this point on, color Doppler and the umbilical pulsations are measurable and quantifiable.

MOUSE

In the mouse, heart tube formation occurs on 8.5 dpc, followed by heart looping on 9.5 dpc, and heart chamber formation on 10.5 dpc. While the heart chambers can be seen via ultrasonography in some fetuses on 10.5 dpc, by 11.5 dpc both chambers are most reliably delineated. Cardiac activity can confirm fetal viability, fetal demise or bradycardia that is concerning for impending fetal demise. At 12.5 dpc, there is distinct separation of the cardiac chambers and by 14.5 dpc the four chambered heart is formed. The umbilical cord is first seen on 9.5 dpc and umbilical cord flow can be detected with pulsations.

Cardiac Anomalies

Recent advances in technology has allowed for detection of some congenital heart defects in the late first trimester, ranging from atrioventricular canal defects, hypoplastic left heart, and transposition of the great arteries (6–8). In mice, from 9.5 to 12.5 dpc, early cardiac formation and function can be detected by ultrasound to confirm that the vascular system has begun development and circulation is present. The detection of congenital heart defects is not readily apparent until at least 13.5 dpc, as the ventricular chamber and outflow tract septation are not completed until 13.5–14.5 dpc (9). Consequently, detection of congenital cardiac anomalies will be most reliably detected in later fetal development stages and are addressed in subsequent chapters. See Figs 2.1–2.4.

LIMB BUDS

Early limb bud and limb formation is very similar across vertebrate species. The limb buds are visible first along the embryonic sides, with establishment of the proximal-distal and anterior-posterior axes. Differing expression of genes results in signals for specific forelimb and hind limb formation (10), and the mesoderm will differentiate into the various tissues of the limb, including the cartilage, bone, muscle, and connective tissue.

HUMAN

In the human between 7 and 8 weeks gestation, the four limbs buds can be seen in the coronal plane, each as small "buds" protruding in a lateral direction from the body At this very early stage, only the beginning development of limb buds is detectable, as the size and growth of the limbs

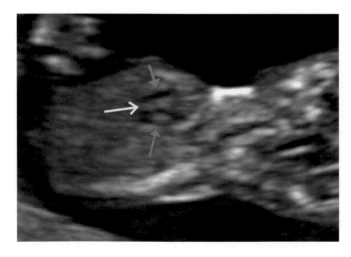

FIGURE 2.1 Earliest detection of the cardiac anatomy, or discrete ventricular structure, occurs from 10 to 11 weeks gestation, as shown above. The cardiac septation (white arrow) between each ventricle (grey arrows) can be clearly seen in these images at 11 weeks gestation. Thus, large anomalies are detectable but smaller, more subtle abnormalities may not be detectable.

(a)   (b)

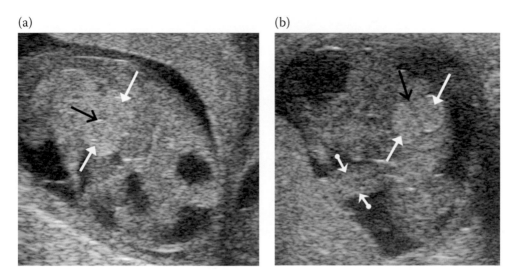

FIGURE 2.2   **A:** In the mouse, on 11.5 dpc, the two chambers of the heart (white arrows) can be distinctly identified within the thorax, as seen her in a sagittal view. **B:** By 12.5 dpc, the two ventricular chambers divided by a muscular septum (black arrow) continue to be readily apparent within the thoracic cavity, appearing as somewhat more echogenic, rounded structures from which a heart rate can be obtained. The two vessels of the umbilical cord are also now visually apparent (short white arrows), leading to the placental site.

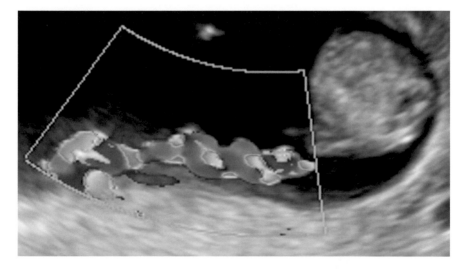

FIGURE 2.3   In the human, at 11 weeks gestation, the arterial and venous flow patterns of the umbilical cord (as depicted by black and grey color flow) are detected. Additionally, the insertion of the umbilical cord into the fetal abdominal wall (white arrow) can be easily detected by color Doppler ultrasound.

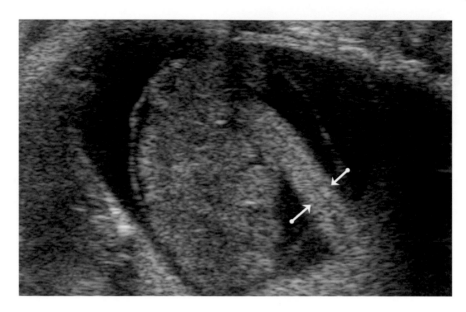

FIGURE 2.4 In the mouse, at 12.5 dpc, the two vessel umbilical cord (each with a white arrow), are shown here with the fetal insertion as well as the placental connection. The localization of the umbilical cord is useful for both detection of maternal and fetal blood flow, as well as localization of the growing placenta.

cannot be reliably quantified. By 9 weeks gestation, the arms and legs elongate and can be seen in the sagittal view. At 10 weeks, the earliest measurements of femur, humerus, tibia, and fibula are detected via transvaginal ultrasound imaging.

MOUSE

The forelimb and hind limb buds are first visible in coronal images of the mouse fetus at 10.5 dpc, and appear in an analogous fashion to human embryos with the appearance of non-elongated "buds" off of the embryonic body, representing mesenchyme condensation. Rapid development from 10.5 to 11.5 dpc results in the appearance of both hind limb tibia and fibula cartilage, in addition to the hind paw. By 12.5 dpc, the limbs have lengthened and developed enough to distinguish upper and lower portions of each limb, as well as the individual digits of paws. Dorsal views of the front paws allow for quantification of "digits" and measurement of length. Of note, hind limbs are morphologically delayed by about half a day, compared to forelimbs.

LIMB ANOMALIES

Major abnormalities in skeletal development and growth such as skeletal dysplasias, achondroplasia, bone malformations, and missing limbs can be detected in early gestational ages (11,12). First trimester ultrasounds provide early identification of missing limb buds and discordant limb growth to elucidate the timing of teratogenic or genetic influences in established mouse models of skeletal disease (13,14). See Figs. 2.5–2.10.

FETAL DEMISE, NORMAL AND ABNORMAL FETAL GROWTH

The earliest quantification methods of fetal growth are obtained through measurements of crown rump length (CRL), which is the linear distance between the top of the head "crown" and the developing

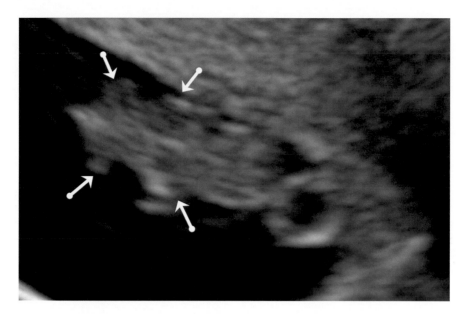

FIGURE 2.5   In the human at 8–10 weeks gestation, the first limb buds are seen, with both the upper arm limb buds easily visualized (white arrows, right), and lower limb buds (white arrows, left) as lateral protrusions from the central axial body and thorax. The buds will continue to elongate, away from the axial skeleton, forming more recognizable limbs.

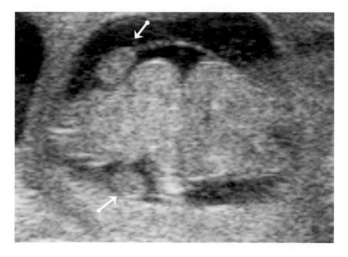

FIGURE 2.6   In the mouse, at 10.5 dpc, the first detection of limb buds is seen, with both hind limb buds visible in the coronal section (white arrows); they are similar and symmetrical in appearance.

buttocks "rump" on ultrasound. The normal interval growth of the human and mouse fetus should follow a predictable pattern, with any lag in growth indicating a concern for an abnormal pregnancy.

HUMAN

Crown rump length (CRL) measurements, in which the distance between the most cephalad and caudal component of the embryo is measured, is routinely used in the first trimester as the standard method of dating pregnancies (15,16). Monitoring the growth of the fetus by CRL allows for the

(a)   (b)

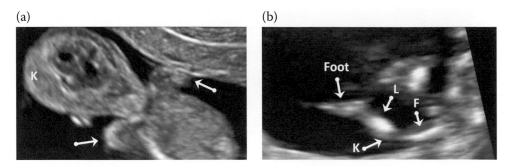

FIGURE 2.7   A: At 11–12 weeks gestation in the human, both shoulders of upper limbs are visible in the coronal plane. The clavicle and scapula have begun ossification by this time. **B:** Also, in this sagittal view the parts of the lower limb are seen, including the foot (F), knee (K), lower leg (L), and femur (F) are visible.

(a)   (b)

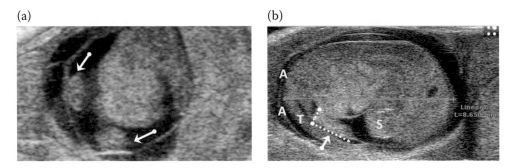

FIGURE 2.8   A: In the mouse, at 11.5 dpc in the transverse view, both forelimb buds are visible, anterior to the chest wall. The limb buds are abutting the clearly visible amniotic membrane. **B:** In the sagittal view, the first view of the hind limb and the hind paw are clearly seen (white arrow pointing to dotted line), between tail (T) and the snout (S). Additionally, the amniotic membrane (A) is easily identified.

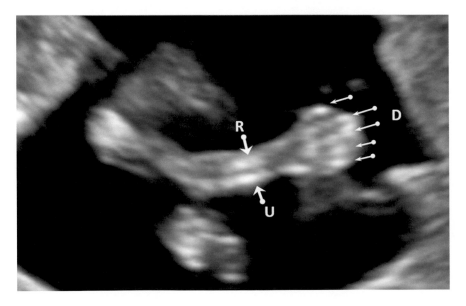

FIGURE 2.9   At 12 weeks in the human, the arm, radius (R), and ulna (U) area easily visualized, in a normally developing right arm. Additionally, at this gestational age, the five digits of the hand (white arrows, D) are able to be observed. At this stage, ossification in the proximal and middle phalanges is now apparent. The ulna measures 9 mm in this measurement.

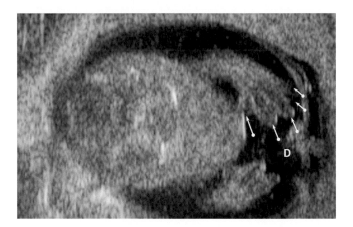

FIGURE 2.10 At 12.5 dpc in the mouse, the forelimb paws hands with digits (white arrows, D) are also easily visualized, and measure at 0.5 mm at this stage. The number and development of each digit can be quantified.

detection of a growth delay during first trimester and is strongly correlated to miscarriage by the end of the first trimester (17,18). Additionally, CRL measurements can help determine embryos which are at risk of having an associated structural congenital anomaly such as major neurological or gastrointestinal structural abnormalities (19).

MOUSE

Mouse models have been extensively used to determine the fetal effects of environmental exposures or genetic abnormalities on fetal growth (cite), as adverse exposures commonly manifest as intrauterine growth restriction. The processes of fetal growth restriction in mice can be established from early pregnancy stages (20).

FIRST TRIMESTER FETAL GROWTH ANOMALIES

Genetically-altered mouse models have proven to be useful and facile tools to determine the genetic contributions of early embryonic development and growth. This allows for mouse models of exposures such as cigarette smoking, alcohol, and medications on fetal growth to be more accurately monitored, documented, and quantified (21,22). The ability to monitor early embryonic growth in the mouse allows for improved data collection, dosage effects, interventions, and specificity of these adverse effects. See Figs. 2.11–2.17.

HEAD AND FACE

The development of craniofacial structures are formed from multiple tissues that unite to form structures of the skull and face. Several prominences give rise to the primary facial structures. The frontonasal (or median nasal) prominence contributes to the forehead, middle of the nose, and the primary palate. The lateral nasal prominence forms the sides of the nose. The maxillomandibular prominences forms the lower jaw and secondary palate. These processes begin and continue throughout the first trimester.

HUMAN

The differentiation of facial tissues occurs early in the embryonic period, between weeks 5 and 7, and the cranium is visible beginning at week 7 and the mandible from weeks 7 to 8. The facial

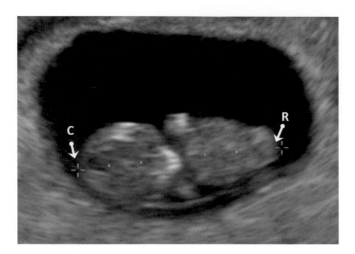

FIGURE 2.11   Human pregnancy with crown (C) rump (R) length at 10 weeks gestation; the polarity of the fetus is visible with the cephalad/"crown" and caudal/"rump" regions easy to determine. The most accurate measurements capture the fetus in the most elongated position possible during the ultrasound.

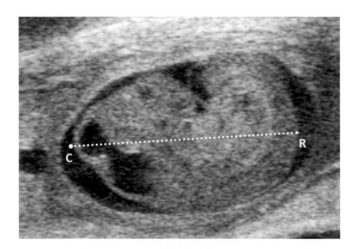

FIGURE 2.12   Mouse pregnancy with crown (C) rump (R) CRL at 10.5 dpc (dotted line); similar to the human, at this point the polarity of the fetus is visible with the cephalad and caudal regions easy to determine. Due to the mouse fetus remaining in a somewhat "curled" position, obtaining an accurate CRL measurement is more reliable, compared to the human fetus at this point.

profile is visible by week 10, due to the ossification of cranial bones during this time (23). In the late first trimester, these features can be seen in a sagittal view and starting at 12 weeks, the fetal secondary palate can be assessed to screen for cleft palate.

MOUSE

Mouse mutants have provided important genetic models for analyzing features that increase probability of spontaneous clefts and increase susceptibility and/or sensitivity to environmentally induced clefts. In the mouse, by 11.5 dpc, the mandible, maxilla and the median nasal process (MNP) – which will become the nose – are developed, and can be appreciated best in the sagittal "profile" view.

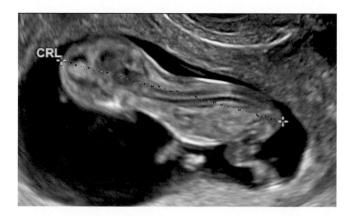

FIGURE 2.13 Human pregnancy with CRL at 11 weeks gestation; the fetus appears more linear at this gestational age and the CRL is measured with the fetus in the most extended position seen. The polarity of the fetus is even more apparent at this gestational age.

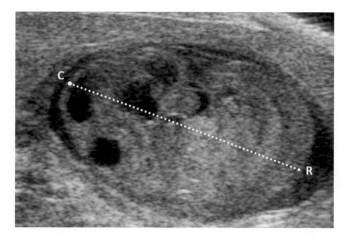

FIGURE 2.14 Mouse pregnancy with crown (C) rump (R) CRL at 11.5 dpc; the mouse fetus still has a more "curled" appearance compared to the human at this stage and a CRL can be easily obtained in a reliable manner. Similarly, the polarity of the fetus is even more apparent at this gestational age.

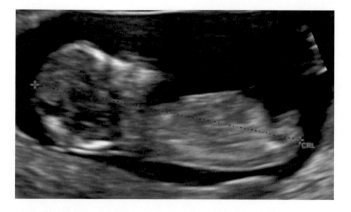

FIGURE 2.15 Human pregnancy with CRL at 12 weeks gestation. In this sagittal or "profile" view, the head begins to take shape with subtle facial features (addressed in detail further in the text). The elongated CRL measurements is seen here being obtained.

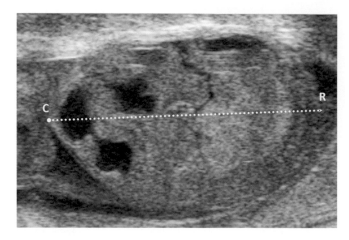

FIGURE 2.16 Mouse pregnancy with crown (C) rump (R) CRL at 12.5 dpc; the difference between the more linear human fetus and the more "curled" mouse fetus is most apparent at this time. The mouse fetus will remain in this position for the entirety of the gestation, while the human fetus will not.

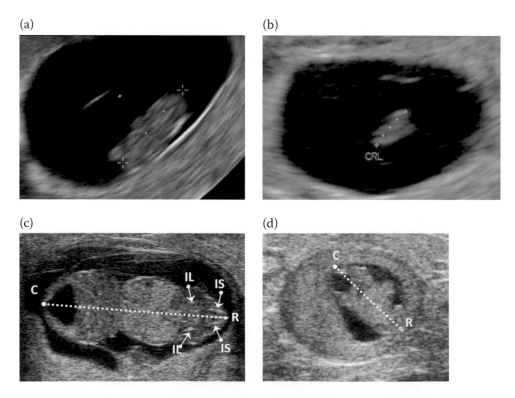

FIGURE 2.17 **A:** A normal human pregnancy at 8 weeks and 6 days, with appropriate interval growth and fetal development, as determined by the CRL measurement. **B:** An abnormal human pregnancy at 8 weeks and 5 days. The CRL measures only at 6 weeks 2 days (5.26 mm) with no fetal cardiac activity seen, confirming a fetal demise. This CRL measurement at this gestational age is not appropriate and lags several weeks behind. **C:** A normal mouse embryo growth on 12.5 dpc, with crown (C) rump (R) CRL measured (dotted line); the ilium (IL), ischium (IS) and base of the tail bones are easily seen in this view. **D:** An abnormal mouse pregnancy at 12.5 dpc. There is lagging, inappropriate fetal growth as determined by the significantly small crown (C) rump (R) CRL measurement, and then confirmed to have no cardiac activity, indicating a fetal demise.

Craniofacial Anomalies

Transgenic mouse models of human disease that result in major craniofacial defects can be more accurately diagnosed and monitored prenatally (24,25), while models of teratogenic exposure such as ethanol that result in facial abnormalities (26) can be monitored in an exposure-stage dependent manner. In humans, early imaging and detection of facial features such as the nasal bone, palate, nose tip, and frontomaxillary facial angle allow early screening for abnormalities such as aneuploidy (27), cleft palate (28) and large craniofacial defects such as holoprosencephaly (25). See Figs. 2.18–2.21.

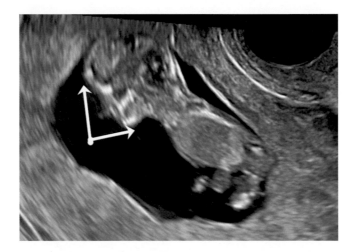

FIGURE 2.18 The human profile (between arrowheads) can begin to be identified between 10 and 11 weeks. At this stage the CRL is approximately 5 cm.

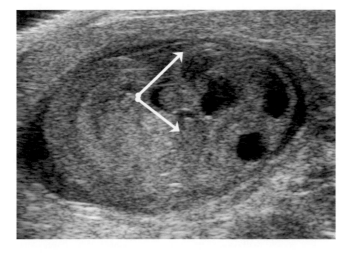

FIGURE 2.19 In the mouse, the earliest gestational time that a profile can be imaged is at 10.5 dpc, with the facial profile seen here (between arrowheads).

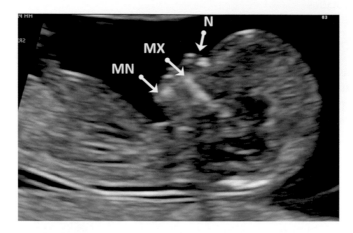

FIGURE 2.20   In the human, after 11 weeks the nasal bridge (N), maxilla (MX) and mandible structures first can be visualized in a profile or sagittal image.

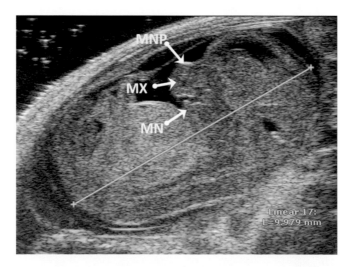

FIGURE 2.21   In the mouse at 12.5 dpc, the mandible, maxilla and the median nasal process (MNP) – which will become the nose – are distinguishable by ultrasound a clear maxilla and mandible are seen in the profile or sagital view. The corresponding fetal size is approximately 10 mm by CRL measurement (grey line).

CHARACTERIZATION OF MULTIFETAL GESTATION AND PREGNANCY SPACING

HUMAN

Human gestations are most often singleton pregnancies. However, multifetal pregnancies such as twin gestations occur, which can be subclassified depending on the presence of shared placenta or amnion; these are designated dichorionic/diamniotic, monochorionic-diamniotic, monochorionic-monoamniotic twins (29). These pregnancies can be most reliably classified by ultrasound after 10–11 weeks. The presence of a "T-sign", which is the inter-twin membrane-placental junction indicates monochorionic-diamniotic twin gestation. Dichorionic twins present with a "lambda sign", where the chorion forms a "wedge-shaped" wall that appears as a curved junction (30).

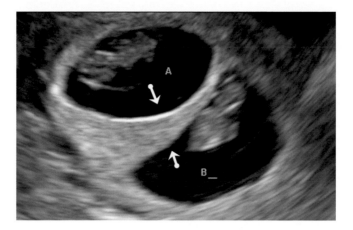

FIGURE 2.22 Human twin gestation at 10 weeks; a dichorionic diamniotic (or "di/di") pregnancy is noted, with a thick septation between (between white arrows) demonstrating the classical "lambda sign".

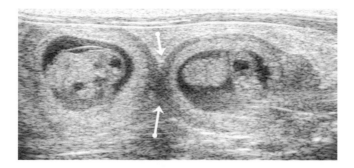

FIGURE 2.23 Mouse pregnancy at 9.5 dpc, demonstrating separation of each gestational sac (between white arrows), as seen in the typical mouse multifetal pregnancy.

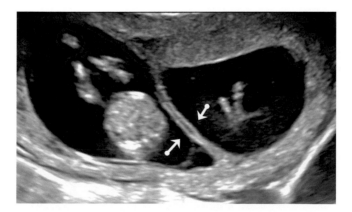

FIGURE 2.24 Human pregnancy at 12 weeks gestation of a dichorionic diamniotic (or "di/di") pregnancy with a thick division (between white arrows) between each fetus.

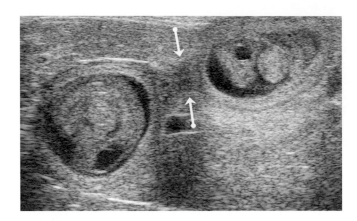

FIGURE 2.25 Mouse pregnancy at 11.5 dpc, with the intervening uterus (between white arrows), which can be seen between each gestational site.

MOUSE

Monozygotic twinning does not occur in mice (31), but all mouse pregnancies (with the exception of severely abnormal phenotypes) have multigestational pregnancies derived from unique zygotes distributed in both uterine horns. Thus, the fetal number, location, and spacing provide valuable information in murine pregnancies. As described previously (Chapter 1), ultrasound can provide this information beginning in early gestation. From 9.5 dpc, the spacing between fetuses can continue to be quantified, with myometrium separating the gestations visible and quantifiable. This can help quantify phenotypes with abnormal embryo spacing (32). See Figs. 2.22–2.25.

REFERENCES

1. Otis, E. M. and Brent, R., Equivalent ages in mouse and human embryos. *Anat Rec.* 1954. 120(1): 33–63.
2. Krishnan, A., Samtani, R., Dhanantwari, P., Lee, E., Yamada, S., Shiota, K., et al., A detailed comparison of mouse and human cardiac development. *Pediatr Res.* 2014. 76(6): 500–507.
3. Moorman, A., Webb, S., Brown, N.A., Lamers, W. and Anderson, R.H., Development of the heart: (1) formation of the cardiac chambers and arterial trunks. *Heart.* 2003. 89(7): 806–814.
4. Hutchinson, D., McBrien, A., Howley, L., Yamamoto, Y., Sekar, P., Motan, T., et al., First-Trimester Fetal Echocardiography: identification of Cardiac Structures for Screening from 6 to 13 Weeks' Gestational Age. *J Am Soc Echocardiogr.* 2017. 30(8): 763–772.
5. Narayan, R., Saaid, R., Pedersen, L. and Hyett, J., Ultrasound assessment of umbilical cord morphology in the first trimester: a feasibility study. *Fetal Diagn Ther.* 2015. 38(3): 212–217.
6. Turan, S., Turan, O. M., Desai, A., Harman, C. R. and Baschat, A.A., First-trimester fetal cardiac examination using spatiotemporal image correlation, tomographic ultrasound and color Doppler imaging for the diagnosis of complex congenital heart disease in high-risk patients. *Ultrasound Obstet Gynecol.* 2014. 44(5): 562–567.
7. Li, Y., Hua, Y., Fang, J., Wang, C., Qiao, L., Wan, C., et al., Performance of different scan protocols of fetal echocardiography in the diagnosis of fetal congenital heart disease: a systematic review and meta-analysis. *PLoS One.* 2013. 8(6): e65484.
8. Liu, H., Zhou, J., Feng, Q. L., Gu, H. T., Wan, G., Zhang, H. M., et al., Fetal echocardiography for congenital heart disease diagnosis: a meta-analysis, power analysis and missing data analysis. *Eur J Prev Cardiol.* 2015. 22(12): 1531–1547.
9. Liu, X., Francis, R., Kim, A. J., Ramirez, R., Chen, G., Subramanian, R., et al., Interrogating congenital heart defects with noninvasive fetal echocardiography in a mouse forward genetic screen. *Circ Cardiovasc Imaging.* 2014. 7(1): 31–42.

10. Shimizu, H., Yokoyama, S. and Asahara, H., Growth and differentiation of the developing limb bud from the perspective of chondrogenesis. *Dev Growth Differ*. 2007. 49(6): 449–454.

11. Fish, E. W., Murdaugh, L. B., Sulik, K. K., Williams, K. P. and Parnell, S. E., Genetic vulnerabilities to prenatal alcohol exposure: limb defects in sonic hedgehog and GLI2 heterozygous mice. *Birth Defects Res*. 2017. 109(11): 860–865.

12. Greene, J. A., Sleet, R. B., Morgan, K. T. and Welsch, F., Cytotoxic effects of ethylene glycol monomethyl ether in the forelimb bud of the mouse embryo. *Teratology*. 1987; 36(1): 23–34.

13. Bird, I. M., Kim, S. H., Schweppe, D. K., Caetano-Lopes, J., Robling, A. G., Charles, J. F., et al., The skeletal phenotype of achondrogenesis type 1A is caused exclusively by cartilage defects. *Development*. 2018. 145(1): 1–13.

14. Lanctot, C., Moreau, A., Chamberland, M., Tremblay, M. L. and Drouin, J., Hindlimb patterning and mandible development require the Ptx1 gene. *Development*. 1999. 126(9): 1805–1810.

15. Napolitano, R., Dhami, J., Ohuma, E. O., Ioannou, C., Conde-Agudelo, A., Kennedy, S. H., et al., Pregnancy dating by fetal crown-rump length: a systematic review of charts. *BJOG*. 2014. 121(5): 556–565.

16. Papageorghiou, A. T., Kennedy, S. H., Salomon, L. J., Ohuma, E. O., Cheikh Ismail, L., Barros, F. C., et al., International standards for early fetal size and pregnancy dating based on ultrasound measurement of crown-rump length in the first trimester of pregnancy. *Ultrasound Obstet Gynecol*. 2014. 44(6): 641–648.

17. Abuelghar, W. M., Fathi, H. M., Ellaithy, M. I. and Anwar, M. A., Can a smaller than expected crown-rump length reliably predict the occurrence of subsequent miscarriage in a viable first trimester pregnancy? *J Obstet Gynaecol Res*. 2013. 39(10): 1449–1455.

18. D'Antonio, F., Khalil, A., Mantovani, E. and Thilaganathan, B., Embryonic growth discordance and early fetal loss: the STORK multiple pregnancy cohort and systematic review. *Hum Reprod*. 2013. 28(10): 2621–2627.

19. Baken, L., Benoit, B., Koning, A. H. J., van der Spek, P. J., Steegers, E. A. P. and Exalto N., First-trimester crown-rump length and embryonic volume of fetuses with structural congenital abnormalities measured in virtual reality: an observational study. *Biomed Res Int*. 2017. 2017: 1953076.

20. Pallares, P. and Gonzalez-Bulnes, A., Intrauterine growth retardation in endothelial nitric oxide synthase-deficient mice is established from early stages of pregnancy. *Biol Reprod*. 2008. 78(6): 1002–1006.

21. Ahmed, A. E., El-Mazar, H. M., Nagy, A. A. and Abdel-Naim, A. B., Chloroacetonitrile induces intrauterine growth restriction and musculoskeletal toxicity in fetal mouse. *Toxicol Ind Health*. 2008. 24(8): 511–518.

22. Mammon, K., Keshet, R., Savion, S., Pekar, O., Zaslavsky, Z., Fein, A., et al., Diabetes-induced fetal growth retardation is associated with suppression of NF-kappaB activity in embryos. *Rev Diabet Stud*. 2005. 2(1): 27–34.

23. Tonni, G., Centini, G. and Rosignoli, L., Prenatal screening for fetal face and clefting in a prospective study on low-risk population: can 3- and 4-dimensional ultrasound enhance visualization and detection rate? *Oral Surg Oral Med Oral Pathol Oral Radiol Endod*. 2005. 100(4): 420–426.

24. Nie, X., Deng, C. X., Wang, Q. and Jiao, K. Disruption of Smad4 in neural crest cells leads to mid-gestation death with pharyngeal arch, craniofacial and cardiac defects. *Dev Biol*. 2008. 316(2): 417–430.

25. Heyne, G. W., Everson, J. L., Ansen-Wilson, L. J., Melberg, C. G., Fink, D. M., Parins, K. F., et al., Gli2 gene-environment interactions contribute to the etiological complexity of holoprosencephaly: evidence from a mouse model. *Dis Model Mech*. 2016. 9(11): 1307–1315.

26. Lipinski, R. J., Hammond, P., O'Leary-Moore, S. K., Ament, J. J., Pecevich, S. J., Jiang, Y., et al., Ethanol-induced face-brain dysmorphology patterns are correlative and exposure-stage dependent. *PLoS One*. 2012. 7(8): e43067.

27. Czuba, B., Cnota, W., Wloch, A., Wegrzyn, P., Sodowski, K., Wielgos, M., et al., Frontomaxillary facial angle measurement in screening for trisomy 18 at 11 + 0 to 13 + 6 weeks of pregnancy: a double-centre study. *Biomed Res Int*. 2013. 2013: 168302.

28. Zajicek, M., Achiron, R., Weisz, B., Shrim, A. and Gindes, L. Sonographic assessment of fetal secondary palate between 12 and 16 weeks of gestation using three-dimensional ultrasound. *Prenat Diagn*. 2013. 33(13): 1256–1259.

29. Hall, J. G., Twinning. *Lancet.* 2003. 362(9385): 735–743.
30. Levy, R., Arfi, J. S., Mirlesse, V. and Jacob, D., Ultrasonic diagnosis of chorionicity in multiple pregnancies. *Gynecol Obstet Fertil.* 2003. 31(11): 960–963.
31. McLaren, A., Molland, P. and Signer, E., Does monozygotic twinning occur in mice? *Genet Res.* 1995. 66(3): 195–202.
32. Lu, S., Peng, H., Zhang, H., Zhang, L., Cao, Q., Li, R., et al., Excessive intrauterine fluid cause aberrant implantation and pregnancy outcome in mice. *PLoS One.* 2013. 8(10): e78446.

3 Mid-Gestation and Second Trimester
Mouse D13.5–15.5; Human 13–27 Weeks

IMAGING

Transabdominal ultrasound imaging can now reliably be used in humans to image the fetus at this gestational age. In mice, the transabdominal approach is continued to be used during this timeframe. Due to the obligate multifetal pregnancies seen in mice, the location of intrauterine pregnancies presents an increased challenge due to crowding of the maternal abdomen. Thus it is recommended that in order to best track individual fetal growth and development, the ultra-sonographer begin each ultrasound at the most proximal site of each uterine horn (the pregnancy located closest to the maternal bladder), and move sequentially down each uterine horn towards the distal end located near the ovary. This will enable more accurate longitudinal tracking of each individual fetus. As at earlier gestational ages, fetal viability thought detection of continued cardiac activity, measurements of fetal growth, and subsequent development of organs can be monitored.

ORGANOGENESIS

In humans, the second trimester is characterized by increased growth and development of organs and systems which were established in the early gestational period. As discussed, mice develop a majority of internal organs between 9.5 and 12.5 dpc, and this chapter will address the additional development of organs from 13.5 onward. This gestational time period allows for a marked increase in the ability to see detailed anatomy and structure of these organ systems in this relatively small animal.

CARDIAC

As reviewed, the development of the cardiac structures in humans and mice are largely quite com-parable (1), allowing the murine cardiac morphogenesis to model human congenital heart disease. At this gestational age in both humans and mice, the four-chambered heart has developed and can be reliably seen on ultrasound in each species (2). Although quite similar, there are a few morphological differences between the species. In the mouse, the left superior cava vena will persist and drain to the coronary sinus; in humans this vessel is replaced by the brachiocephalic vein, which is connected to a right-sided superior vena cava (3). Transgenic mouse models have been widely used to determine genetic variants attributable to human and mouse cardiac development during this gestational stage (4,5) and thousands of transgenic mouse models with cardiac anomalies have been identified (3).

HUMAN

The fetal heart is completely formed by approximately 8 weeks gestation, however the ventricular structures and outflow tracts cannot be visualized at this early time point; by the 11th week gestation the four chambers of the heart can be detected (6), in addition to larger congenital malformations (7). Ultrasound at during the second trimester can detect congenital heart disease in approximately 80–90% in pregnancies with an elevated risk of congenital anomalies; however routine screening for low risk populations is not recommended (8,9).

MOUSE

In the mouse, on 8.5 dpc heart tube formation occurs, followed by heart looping on 9.5 dpc, and heart chamber formation on 10.5 dpc. While the heart chambers can be seen via ultrasonography in some fetuses on 10.5 dpc, by 11.5 dpc both chambers are most reliably visualized and delineated. Cardiac structures within the thorax can be seen in relaxation and constriction phases, confirming either fetal viability, fetal demise or bradycardia that is concerning for impending fetal demise. By the time of 12.5 dpc, there is distinct separation of the cardiac chambers; by 14.5 dpc four chambered heart is formed. From 13.5 to 15.5, continued cardiac development and function can be

(a)   (b)

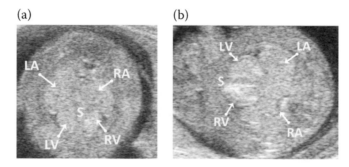

FIGURE 3.1   AB: D13.5 – The four chambers of the heart can now be appreciated on 13.5 dpc. In a transverse view of the thorax, as seen in each of the representative images, the left atrium (LA), right atrium (RA), left ventricle (LV) and right ventricle (RV) are appreciated. The septal wall (S) dividing the ventricles is also apparent. Two examples of the cardiac structures are provided.

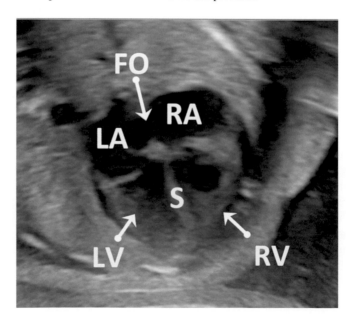

FIGURE 3.2   At 18 weeks gestation, the four chambers of the human heart are easily discernible. The left atrium (LA), right atrium (RA), foramen ovale (FO) left ventricle (LV) and right ventricle (RV) are appreciated. The septal wall (S) dividing the ventricles is also apparent.

monitored by ultrasound more reliably compared to earlier gestational age, due primarily to the increase in cardiac size. These factors allow for the routine detection of congenital heart defects beginning 13.5 dpc, when critical events such as ventricular chamber and outflow tract septation are completed (3,10). The septation of the common outflow tract contributes to the formation of outlets, valves, and bases of the aortic and pulmonary trunks at 13.5 dpc (3).

Cardiac Anomalies

Congenital heart disease has an estimated incidence of 1% of live births, with a large majority of congenital anomalies considered to be due to a multifactorial developmental background (5). It has been suspected that cardiac anomalies may be the underlying cause for up to 60–80% of early embryonic in some of the earlier knockout transgenic mouse studies (11). See Figs. 3.1–3.6.

(a)   (b)

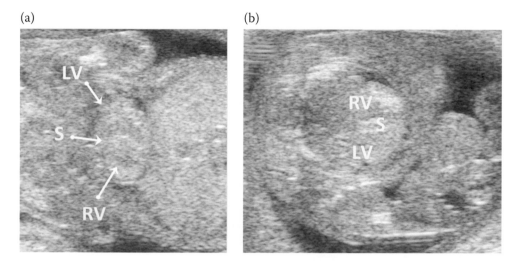

FIGURE 3.3   AB: D14.5 – heart chambers of the heart, including the ventricular septum (S) continue to develop, as seen dividing both the ventricle (LV) and right ventricle (RV). The atrial septum is not appreciable at this gestational age. The myocardium of each ventricle is seen as a brighter/more echogenic structure with the blood (darker) filling the ventricle.

(a)   (b)

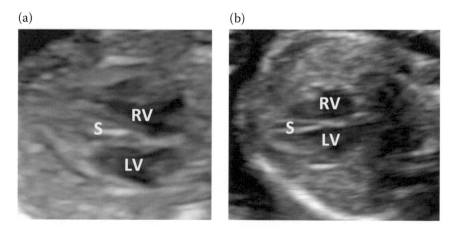

FIGURE 3.4   AB: In this plane, the right and left ventricles of the human heart are seen, with the septum separating the left ventricle (LV) and right ventricle (RV). The entire length of the septal wall (S) dividing the ventricles is able to be seen, extending to the apex of the heart.

(a)   (b)

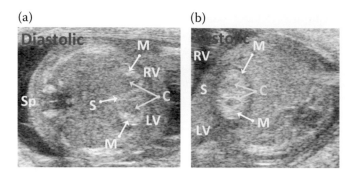

FIGURE 3.5 **AB:** D15.5 – at this gestational age, the increased growth of the cardiac structures, most notably the ventricles, allows for the systolic and diastolic states to be easily distinguished. The above images are of the right ventricle (RV) and the left ventricle (LV) in both the relaxed and contractile states. The myocardium (M) of each ventricle is seen as a brighter/more echogenic structure with the blood (darker) filling the chamber (C) of each ventricle. The vertebral bodies of the spine (Sp) indicates the posterior aspect of the fetus; the heart is located in the anterior portion of the thorax.

(a)   (b)

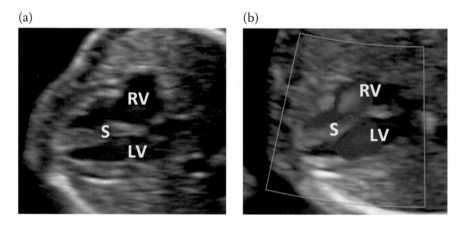

FIGURE 3.6 **AB:** During the second trimester, the long-axis view of the left (LV) and right (RV) ventricles are able to be obtained. With the assistance of color flow Doppler, blood flow within each ventricle as well as the dividing ventricular septum (S) are easily demarcated (as shown in B).

DIAPHRAGM

OVERVIEW

The diaphragm is a muscle required for respiration and defects in its development can lead to severe anomalies such as congenital diaphragmatic hernias (CDH) (12). These birth defects are not uncommon birth defects and result in severe morbidity or mortality, thus detecting the normal or abnormal development during gestational is of critical importance.

Human

The diaphragm forms in the human between the seventh and 12th week of pregnancy. Confirming intact diaphragms on each side is best when assessed posteriorly near the spine, which is a common site for diaphragmatic abnormalities and will have a clear curvilinear separation if anatomy is normal. The lungs will appear as lighter and more homogeneous compared to the fetal abdominal contents. The diaphragm begins functioning in utero, and in the third trimester preparatory detectable fetal respiratory movements or "breathing" occurs, which are posited to have a several roles in development.

Mouse

The development of the fetal mouse diaphragm begins at approximately 8.5 dpc with the formation of the septum transversum (13). A rapid increase in the presence of somites and muscle within the diaphragm occurs in the mouse from 12.5 dpc to 13.5 dpc; it is at this time point the diaphragm is able to be visualized in the mouse fetal via ultrasound (13). Of note, while human fetal respiratory movements are seen on ultrasound in the third trimester, the mouse fetus does not exhibit respiratory movements that are detectable by ultrasound technology.

Diaphragm Anomalies

The mouse has been used successfully as a model for human diaphragmatic diseases (14,15), including hypoplasia and congenital diaphragmatic hernias (CDH) congenital malformations (16). Recent screening of genes expressed in the development of the mouse diaphragm identified a list of 27 candidate CDH-causing genes (17), exemplifying the utility of mouse models in translational research. As CDH develops prior to 12.5 dpc in mouse models (18), this suggests that at 13.5 dpc, when the fetal mouse diaphragm is first reliably detected via ultrasound, significant diaphragmatic abnormalities will be detectable. See Figs. 3.7–3.10.

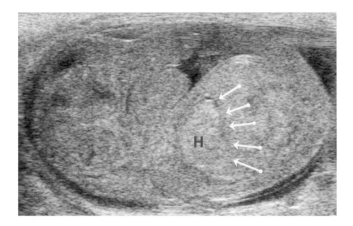

FIGURE 3.7 D13.5 – The diaphragm is first identified via ultrasound at gestational age of 13.5 dpc in the mouse fetus. In this sagittal plane view, the diaphragm is seen as a darker, linear line (white arrow tips) dividing the heart (H) within the thorax.

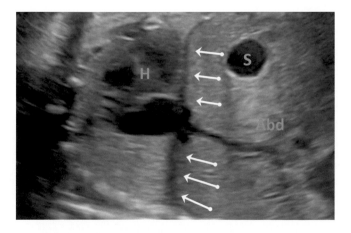

FIGURE 3.8 During mid gestation, the diaphragm can be routinely identified. Similar to the mouse, the human diaphragm is a darker, linear line (white arrow tips) dividing the heart (H) within the thorax and the intestines within the abdominal cavity (Abd). The stomach (S) can also be seen in this view.

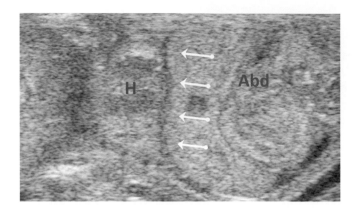

FIGURE 3.9   D15.5 – With the continued growth of the fetus, the location of the heart (H) above the diaphragm remains clear. The dark, curvilinear line of the diaphragmatic muscle is easy to identify, separating the thoracic cavity from the abdominal cavity (Abd).

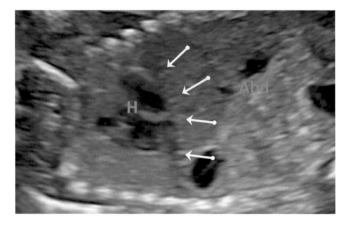

FIGURE 3.10   The human fetal diaphragm still appears very similar to the mouse diaphragm in orientation. The human diaphragm is a linear line (white arrow tips) dividing the heart (H) within the thorax and the intestines within the abdominal cavity (Abd).

EXTREMITIES

The continued limb and skeletal formation processes are similar among vertebrate lineages (19). The human and mouse extremities are quite analogous, with similar development and function (20); thus ultrasound can be used to assess limb length and identify skeletal malformations, even at this mid-gestational age.

HUMAN

Structures such as the long bones will ossify by 11–12 weeks of gestation, and are expected to be consistently seen after 12 weeks on ultrasound (21). The metacarpals and metatarsals are ossified by 12–16 weeks. A normal fetal hand can be seen at 18 weeks gestation (22). Severe limb reductions can be detected by femur length at 16–18 weeks of gestation, but some more moderate or mild forms of limb abnormalities such as achondroplasia may not become obvious until 22–24 weeks (23).

MOUSE

At 11.5 the humerus is beginning to form, with rapid growth occurring so that by 14.5 the most distal phalanges of the forepaw are shaped (24). Of note, the human thumb is analogous to the mouse pollex, which is a very short protrusion with a nail and not a fully elongated digit. In the mouse, the ossification of humerus and femur occur first, followed by the radius/ulna and tibia and fibula, and lastly the digits. Resultantly, on ultrasound these bony structures are first detectable in this order (25).

PAW AND HAND ANOMALIES

Malformations of the hand include clenched hand, thumb anomalies, abnormal size, or abnormal number (polydactyly, syndactyly, ectrodactyly). These malformations can be isolated but are often associated with a syndrome or chromosomal anomaly (26). Mouse models with genetic mutations have demonstrated abnormalities such as syndactyly and postaxial polydactyly (27), with a majority of the transgenic mouse research elucidating he role of bone morphogenetic proteins (BMP) in limb and paw development (28). See Figs. 3.11–3.18.

LONG BONE AND LIMB ANOMALIES

Progressive maturation of the bones occurs at specific time points. At 14.5 dpc, the chondrocytes in the center of the mouse tibia will undergo progressive maturation, allowing for reliable ultrasound detection of the lower hind limb bone structures (29). Thus, mouse models of abnormal limb growth and dwarfism can show difference as early as 14.5 dpc (30). Genetically modified mice

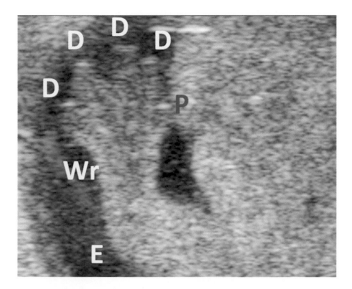

FIGURE 3.11   D13.5 – At this gestational age, significant apoptosis occurs between the fetal mouse digits of the paw, resulting in individual elongated digits. The mouse forepaw has five digits, including small pollex (P) with a flattened nail which is found on the medial portion of the forepaw (analogous to the human thumb). Each digit (D) is seen in the image, with additional forearm anatomy of the wrist (Wr) and elbow (E) visible.

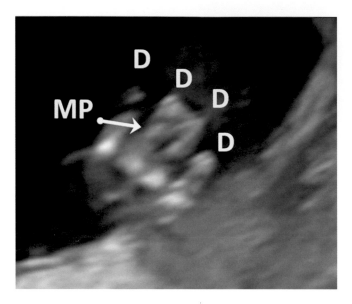

FIGURE 3.12 The ossified distal and middles phalanges (MP) of the hand can be easily appreciated during the second trimester. Coronal sonogram of the hand demonstrating some of the bony detail of the developing phalanges with the middle phalanx (MP) highlighted. Unlike the mouse, the human hand is often clenched in a fist, which can make the counting of digits more difficult.

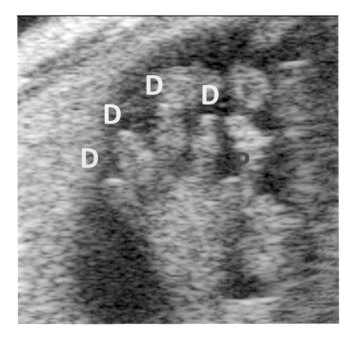

FIGURE 3.13 D14.5 – By 14.5 dpc in the mouse, interdigitary apoptosis has allowed for individual digits (D) and the pollex (P) to be appreciated. Unlike the human, whose hand is most often seen in a clenched manner, the mouse paw is more frequently observed in the open position. This allows for the number, size, and position of each mouse digit to be clearly characterized, perhaps even more so than the human.

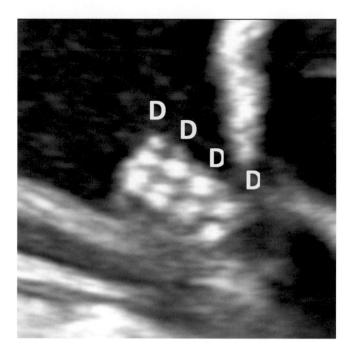

FIGURE 3.14 In the human during the second trimester, the gaps between the ends of bones are filled with cartilage, which are seen as a light grey area between the echogenic appearances of the hard, ossified bone. The four phalanges of the digits (D) and thumb (T) are visible; the thumb is analogous to the mouse pollex digit, being both the shortest digit and located on the radial side of the hand.

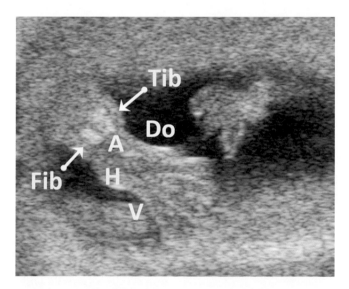

FIGURE 3.15 In the mouse at 14.5 dpc, the hind limb paw, which is analogous to the human foot, begins to take shape via ultrasonographic findings. The image demonstrates the orientation of the hind limb paw, including the dorsal (Do) and ventral (V) aspects of the paw. Additionally, the ossified centers of the lower leg bones tibia (T) and fibula (F), the ankle (A), heel (H) and are all appreciable.

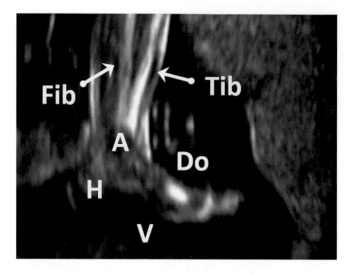

FIGURE 3.16   The human foot can be viewed in an analogous manner to the mouse hind paw. In this image, every analogous structure that is seen in the mouse at 14.5 dpc can also be detected in the human. The ossified centers of the lower leg bones tibia (T) and fibula (F), the ankle (A) and the ventral (V) and dorsal (D) aspects of the human leg and foot are all appreciable in a similar orientation to the fetal mouse.

(a)   (b)

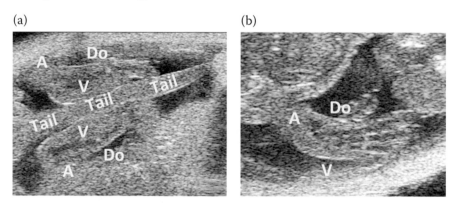

FIGURE 3.17   AB: D15.5 – the structures of the hind limb paw are analogous to the human foot. In A, the ankle (A), and the ventral (V) and dorsal (Do) regions of the paw are seen, with tail (T) between them. The ossified bones of the feet can first be reliably detected and counted on 15.5 dpc in the mouse embryo.

(a)   (b)

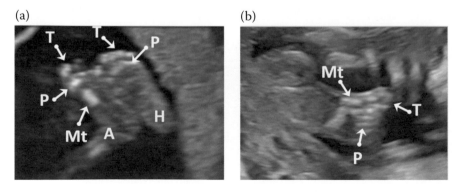

FIGURE 3.18   The fetal foot at 18 weeks gestation in the transverse axial (A) and parasagittal (B) planes are represented. In these images, the toes (T), proximal phalangeal ossification centers (P) and the metatarsal ossification centers (Mt) are visible. While most of the foot and hind limb paw anatomy are similar, one important difference to note is the relative lengths of each toe. In the mouse, the three central toes are of similar length, while the lateral and medial toes are equally short.

(a)   (b)

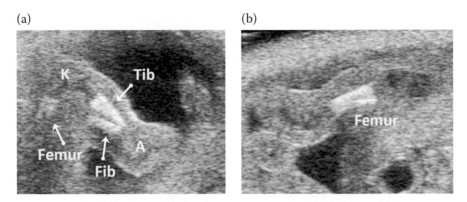

FIGURE 3.19   AB: D14.5 – At this time, the tibia (Tib), fibula (Fib) and the femur can be measured. The ossified bone will appear as bright white and echogenic, while the cartilage appears as a lighted gray, making it difficult to detect from nearby soft tissues that occurs in the knee (K) and ankle (A) joints. The ossified bones of the mouse are still very small at the gestational age; for perspective, in A the fibula measures 0.8 mm and the tibia measures 1.0 mm. In B, the length of the femur is measured at 1.1 mm.

(a)   (b)

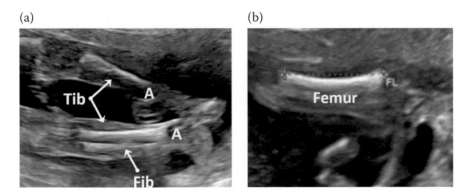

FIGURE 3.20   AB: The long bones of the human lower extremity remain analogous to the mouse at this gestational age. When positioned in the correct plane, ultrasound can provide the length of the tibia (Tib), fibula (Fib) and femur, just as simply as the mouse fetus at 15.5 dpc.

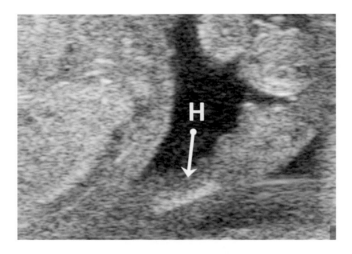

FIGURE 3.21   D14.5 – The best images of the elongated humerus are found by using a transverse view of the abdomen or thorax to obtain the best plain and longest measurement of the bone; for scale and proportion, the ossified portion of the humerus at this gestational age in the mouse is measured between 0.9 and 1.0 mm.

with abnormal musculature have allowed for modeling of abnormal muscle contractions on mammalian bone development (31). Achondroplasia has been modeled by transgenic mouse models (32); performing sequential fetal ultrasounds can provide fetal growth parameters as well. See Figs. 3.19–3.24.

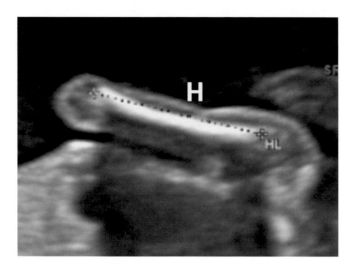

FIGURE 3.22   During mid gestation in the human, the humerus (H) can easily be measured in its longest dimension, with the view of the upper arm at the side of the thorax in the coronal or frontal plane. Notably, this plane is different compared to the mouse, in which a transverse plan offers the best view of the humerus at this gestational time point.

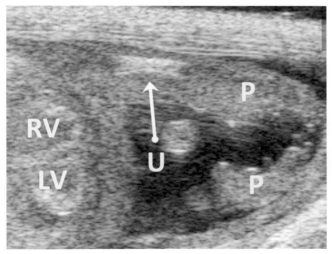

FIGURE 3.23   D15.5 – The ulna of the upper limb is measurable, however the radius is not as easily detected at this gestational age. The forelimb paw (P) are labeled; the ulna and the forelimb paws are anterior to the thorax and abdomen, with the pads of the paw (analogous to the human palm) facing each other in the medial plane. The image incidentally provides a transverse cross section of the left and right ventricles (LV, RV).

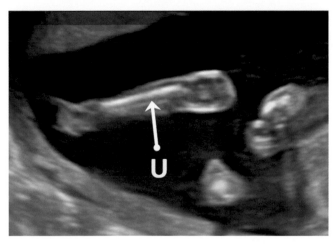

FIGURE 3.24 The human upper extremity long bones are more apparent compared to the mouse during this mid gestational period. The size and growth of the human fetus allows for both the ulna (U) and the radius to be detected and measured, unlike the mouse in which the ulna is by far a more reliable finding.

REFERENCES

1. Krishnan, A., Samtani, R., Dhanantwari, P., Lee, E., Yamada, S., Shiota, K., Donofrio, M. T., Leatherbury, L. and Lo, C.W., A detailed comparison of mouse and human cardiac development. *Pediatr Res*, 2014. 76(6): 500–507.
2. Moorman, A., et al., Development of the heart: (1) formation of the cardiac chambers and arterial trunks. *Heart*, 2003. 89(7): 806–814.
3. Savolainen, S. M., Foley, J. F. and Elmore, S. A., Histology atlas of the developing mouse heart with emphasis on E11.5 to E18.5. *Toxicol Pathol*, 2009. 37(4): 395–414.
4. Gittenberger-de Groot, A. C., et al., Basics of cardiac development for the understanding of congenital heart malformations. *Pediatr Res*, 2005. 57(2): 169–176.
5. Gittenberger-de Groot, A. C., et al., Embryology of the heart and its impact on understanding fetal and neonatal heart disease. *Semin Fetal Neonatal Med*, 2013. 18(5): 237–244.
6. Hutchinson, D., et al., First-trimester fetal echocardiography: identification of cardiac structures for screening from 6 to 13 weeks' Gestational Age. *J Am Soc Echocardiogr*, 2017. 30(8): p. 763–772.
7. Markou, G. A., Dafereras, G. and Poncelet, C., Congenital cystic adenomatoid malformation diagnosed during first-trimester ultrasound scan. *Am J Case Rep*, 2018. 19: 1–4.
8. Randall, P., et al., Accuracy of fetal echocardiography in the routine detection of congenital heart disease among unselected and low risk populations: a systematic review. *BJOG*, 2005. 112(1): 24–30.
9. Zhang, Y. F., et al., Diagnostic value of fetal echocardiography for congenital heart disease: a systematic review and meta-analysis. *Medicine (Baltimore)*, 2015. 94(42): e1759.
10. Liu, X., et al., Interrogating congenital heart defects with noninvasive fetal echocardiography in a mouse forward genetic screen. *Circ Cardiovasc Imaging*, 2014. **7**(1): 31–42.
11. Brandon, E. P., Idzerda, R. L. and McKnight, G.S., Targeting the mouse genome: a compendium of knockouts (Part II). *Curr Biol*, 1995. 5(7): 758–765.
12. Merrell, A. J. and Kardon, G., Development of the diaphragm – a skeletal muscle essential for mammalian respiration. *FEBS J*, 2013. 280(17): 4026–4035.
13. Kardon, G., et al., Congenital diaphragmatic hernias: from genes to mechanisms to therapies. *Dis Model Mech*, 2017. 10(8): 955–970.
14. Ackerman, K. G. and Greer, J. J., Development of the diaphragm and genetic mouse models of diaphragmatic defects. *Am J Med Genet C Semin Med Genet*, 2007. 145C(2): 109–116.
15. Paris, N. D., Coles, G. L. and Ackerman, K. G., Wt1 and beta-catenin cooperatively regulate diaphragm development in the mouse. *Dev Biol*, 2015. 407(1): 40–56.
16. You, L. R., et al., Mouse lacking COUP-TFII as an animal model of Bochdalek-type congenital diaphragmatic hernia. *Proc Natl Acad Sci U S A*, 2005. 102(45): 16351–16356.
17. Russell, M. K., et al., Congenital diaphragmatic hernia candidate genes derived from embryonic transcriptomes. *Proc Natl Acad Sci U S A*, 2012. 109(8): 2978–2983.
18. Sefton, E. M., Gallardo, M. and Kardon, G., Developmental origin and morphogenesis of the diaphragm, an essential mammalian muscle. *Dev Biol*, 2018. 440(2): 64–73.

19. Giffin, J. L., Gaitor, D. and Franz-Odendaal, T. A., The forgotten skeletogenic condensations: a comparison of early skeletal development amongst vertebrates. *J Dev Biol*, 2019. 7(1).

20. Chang, S. H., et al., Comparison of mouse and human ankles and establishment of mouse ankle osteoarthritis models by surgically-induced instability. *Osteoarthritis Cartilage*, 2016. 24(4): 688–697.

21. Noel, A. E. and Brown, R. N., Advances in evaluating the fetal skeleton. *Int J Womens Health*, 2014. 6: 489–500.

22. D'Ambrosio, V., et al., Midtrimester isolated short femur and perinatal outcomes: A systematic review and meta-analysis. *Acta Obstet Gynecol Scand*, 2019. 98(1): 11–17.

23. Krakow, D., et al., Mutations in the gene encoding the calcium-permeable ion channel TRPV4 produce spondylometaphyseal dysplasia, Kozlowski type and metatropic dysplasia. *Am J Hum Genet*, 2009. 84(3): 307–315.

24. Martin, P., Tissue patterning in the developing mouse limb. *Int J Dev Biol*, 1990. 34(3): 323–336.

25. Rafipay, A., et al., Expression analysis of limb element markers during mouse embryonic development. *Dev Dyn*, 2018. 247(11): 1217–1226.

26. Stoll, C., et al., Evaluation of the prenatal diagnosis of limb reduction deficiencies. EUROSCAN Study Group. *Prenat Diagn*, 2000. 20(10): 811–818.

27. Wang, C. K., et al., Function of BMPs in the apical ectoderm of the developing mouse limb. *Dev Biol*, 2004. 269(1): 109–122.

28. Robert, B., Bone morphogenetic protein signaling in limb outgrowth and patterning. *Dev Growth Differ*, 2007. 49(6): 455–468.

29. Long, F. and Ornitz, D. M., Development of the endochondral skeleton. *Cold Spring Harb Perspect Biol*, 2013. 5(1): a008334.

30. Kato, K., et al., SOXC transcription factors induce cartilage growth plate formation in mouse embryos by promoting noncanonical WNT signaling. *J Bone Miner Res*, 2015. 30(9): 1560–1571.

31. Nowlan, N. C., et al., Mechanobiology of embryonic skeletal development: insights from animal models. *Birth Defects Res C Embryo Today*, 2010. 90(3): 203–213.

32. Lee, Y. C., et al., Knock-in human FGFR3 achondroplasia mutation as a mouse model for human skeletal dysplasia. *Sci Rep*, 2017. 7: 43220.

4 Central Nervous System and Facial Development
Mouse D13.5–15.5; Human 13–27 Weeks

In mice, the first two trimesters of development are considered to include 0.5–E14.5 or 15.5; the "last trimester" actually extends after 15.5 dpc to the 10th post-natal day after birth. Thus, as portion of the later development of the mouse in this "third trimester" includes developments that occur after birth (1) and will not be demonstrated in these images. This later gestational age has been chosen to demonstrate CNS and facial comparisons, as these images are most easily obtained in mice and humans.

IMAGING OF CENTRAL NERVOUS SYSTEM AND FACIAL DEVELOPMENT

In both humans and mice, obtaining images of CNS as the face rely on accurate positioning and obtaining the correct plane of the ultrasound probe to the fetus. For facial imaging of the nose, lips and mouth, the frontal plan can best offer these images. The imaging of the spinal cord and tail often will not be obtained in one frame; thus, multiple images will need to be obtained. The brain structure also will need to be obtained in multiple planes.

CENTRAL NERVOUS SYSTEM AND FACIAL DEVELOPMENT

In humans, the standard imaging techniques for the fetal brain include the biparietal diameter, transventricular plane and the cerebellar planes. The sagittal images of the brain can include the mid line brain structures, the coronal face views, and the coronal cerebellum views. The fetal face can be analyzed in both the axial and coronal views; from these images the size and spacing of the eyes as well as the upper lip are identified. During this timeframe the first images of the face are obtained, showing distinct facial structures.

NASAL STRUCTURES AND PALATE

The development of the face in both humans and mice is an intricate process. The roof of the mouth is formed by the palate, which serves to separate the nasal and oral cavities. For both humans and mice, the palate is formed from both the primary and the secondary palates. The primary palate is the most anterior part of the palate, while the secondary palate – which creates the majority of the palate – forms by a process of fusion of two paired palatal shelves, which are derived from the maxillary processes (2,3).

HUMAN

The formation of the palate occurs in the first trimester, but is unable to be assessed via ultrasound until the second trimester. The palatal shelves fuse and form an intact palate at approximately 9 weeks gestation (2–4). On ultrasound, a coronal view of the nose (with two nostrils), upper lip, lower lip, and chin should be visible in the same coronal plane. The midsagittal plane or "profile" allows for the view of forehead, nose, and jaw; ultrasounds performed during the midtrimester often allow for the best imaging, before fetal growth and crowding obscures accurate views (5–7).

MOUSE

The secondary palate begins development at 11.5 dpc as with the palatal shelf outgrowths arising from the oral surface of the maxillary processes, followed by vertical growth which forms the palatal shelves (8). At 13.5 dpc the palatal shelves can are now distinct forms along the anterior-posterior axis. Of note, the most critical coordination of events occur from 14.0 to 15.5 dpc in the mouse fetus. Elevation of the palatal shelves occurs in the short time frame from 14–14.5 dpc, followed by contact of the palatal shelves at 15.0 dpc. After meeting in the midline, the palatal shelves will completion of fusion of the palate by 15.5 dpc (8,9); these above actions correlate to palatogenesis events beginning in the sixth week of gestation with completion of palatal fusion by 12 weeks (8).

ANOMALIES

Facial clefts, including cleft lip with or without cleft palate, are the second most common congenital malformation (10). Typical facial defects are commonly thought to occur from failure of fusion of the different bony processes and overlying soft tissue structure. The etiology of these defects is likely a combination of genetics and environmental exposures during embryologic development. Mouse models have now been applied widely to discover the causes and pathogenesis of cleft palate (8,9), and numerous genes have also been implicated which have with wide-ranging cellular functions (11). See Figs. 4.1–4.4.

EYE

The development of the eye occurs early in the embryological process in both humans and mice. Both species follow a similar developmental process and pattern, with both mouse and human possessing a

(a)   (b)

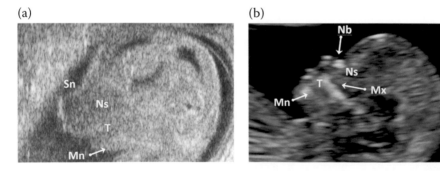

FIGURE 4.1 A: D13.5 – The first time that a reliable profile of the mouse can be obtained is at 13.5 dpc. In this sagittal or profile view, midline structures such as the nasal septum (Ns), tongue (T), and the mandible (Mn) can be visualized via ultrasound. The shape of the snout (Sn) can be appreciated in profile. **B:** At 14 weeks gestation in humans, the sagittal/profile view permits visualization of analogous structures that are found in the mouse at this developmental age. Facial structures such as the nasal bone (Nb), nose tip (Nt) tongue (T), mandible (Mn), and maxilla (Mx) are seen in this view. The full length of the echogenic calcified nasal bone can be measured at this gestational age; a hypoplastic nasal bone has been associated with an increased risk of Trisomy 21. The mouse does not have an ossified structural correlate detected on ultrasound as easily as human nasal bone, although the shape of the snout is seen in profile.

(a)

(b)

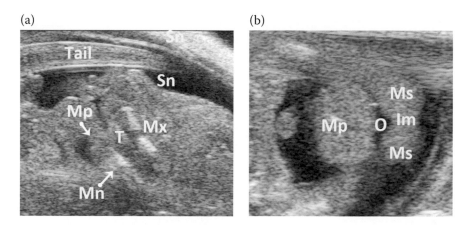

FIGURE 4.2 15.5 dpc – the sagittal plane (A) allows the structures to be visualized in profile; the mouse fetal snout elongates and the maxillary bones are more echogenic. The tail (T) of the mouse is folded under the ventral plane, extending in front of the face. The mandible (Mn), maxilla (Mx) and oral cavity (O) are all captured in the same plan. In the frontal/coronal plane (B), the mandibular prominence (Mp), oral cavity (O), and the maxillary prominence (Mp) are distinguished. These are analogous to the commonly obtained frontal view of the human nose and lips.

(a)

(b)

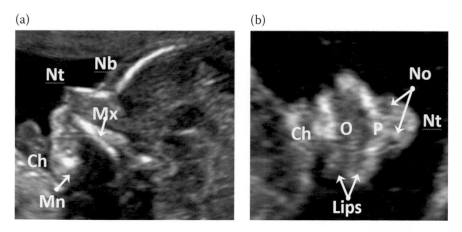

FIGURE 4.3 (A) The sagittal view, similar to the mouse profile, demonstrates the mandible (Mn), maxilla (Mx) and oral cavity are all captured in the same plan. The ossified nasal bone is seen. (B) A coronal image of the nose and upper lip can demonstrate the structures of the nose tip (Nt) nostril (No), upper and lower lips (Lips), philtrum (P), oral cavity (O) and mandibular prominence or chin (Ch). Nostrils of the human are seen at this age, but not the nostrils of the mouse.

lens, vitreous humor, retina, and posterior retinal, optic nerve, cornea, and lids. One primary difference in the species is that in mice, eyes are closed at birth and then open around post-natal day 14.

HUMAN

In early development, the eyes are lateral and migrate medially as gestation continues; both the orbit as well as the lens of the eye are seen via ultrasound. The lenses are seen as central circles that do not have internal echogenicity, first seen around 13 weeks gestation (12). Distance between the orbits are usually taken in an axial plane, with abnormal distance correlating to hyper or hypo-telorism.

(a)   (b)

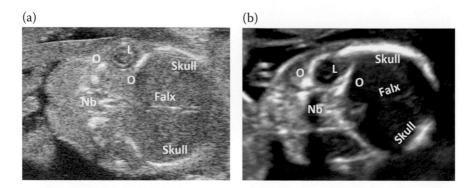

FIGURE 4.4 A: D15.5 coronal plane – at 15.5 dpc, the distinct bones of the skull, orbits (O), and nasal bone (Nb) are seen in this view. The ossified bones of the skull are visible (with the division between the hemispheres seen in each). This view also allows for eye structures such as the orbit (O) and lens (L) to be seen easily in both the mouse and human. The falx cerebri (Falx) is seen in the midline brain. **B:** The facial bone structure of the human is quite analogous to the mouse at this gestational age. The skull, orbits, bones of the midface, including the nasal bone (Nb) are seen in this cross-sectional view. Similar to the mouse, the ossified bones of the skull are visible (with the division between the hemispheres demarcated by the falx cerebri (Falx). The similarities in the development and morphology of mouse and anatomy are quite apparent.

Mouse

Similar to the human, the axial plane allows for the spacing of the orbits to be measured. Via ultrasound, retinal development is apparent beginning at 13.5 dpc, as the posterior lens demonstrates a thickening its echogenic border. The corneal development is first seen at 14.5 dpc, with the anterior and posterior surfaces of the cornea measuring approximately 120 µm. Additionally, at 14.5 dpc, the developing vitreous cavity is easily seen immediately posterior to the lens, followed by the echoic retina (13). The biorbital distance is also measurable beginning at 13.5 dpc.

Anomalies

Numerous orbital anomalies can be detected. Hypertelorism and hypotelorism are detected my measuring the distance between the orbits during midgestation, which are often associated with other anomalies as part of a syndrome. Numerous mouse models with known genetic mutations have resulted in congenital hypertelorism (14–16). Congenital cataracts are identified as echogenicity of the lens, and can be detected between 13 and 27 weeks gestation (12,17). Other mouse models have offered techniques to study human ocular diseases such as cataracts, glaucoma, retinoblastoma, congenital cataracts, and intraocular tumors (12,18–20). See Figs. 4.5–4.6.

SPINE

The formation of the neural tube, which will become the brain and spinal cord, begins in the first trimester, although abnormalities cannot be reliably detected via ultrasound until the second trimester (21). The neural plate is formed and undergoes elongation, followed by elevation of lateral borders into the neural folds which fuse in the midline. In both mice and humans, the spinal cord is contained within the bony vertebrae, which is characterized by regions of cervical, thoracic, lumbar, and the fused sacral and coccyx vertebrae.

(a)   (b)

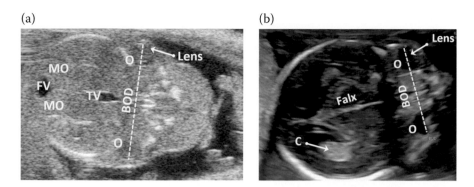

FIGURE 4.5 A: D14.5 – in the transaxial plane, the eye, lens, retina, and the biorbital distance (BOD) are able to be measured in the mouse in a very analogous manner to the human fetal measurement. The BOD is a common measurement obtained in human antenatal ultrasounds. At 13.5 dpc, the BOD measures 3.8 mm and in this example, at 14.5 dpc, the BOD measures 0.44 cm. Additional central nervous system structures in this plane include, fourth ventricle (FV), medulla oblongata (MO), and the third ventricle (TV). **B:** During the second trimester, similar ocular structures are visible in the human, including orbit (O) and lens of the eye (L). For comparison, the BOD in the human measures 3.2 cm compared to 0.44 cm as seen in the mouse.

(a)   (b)

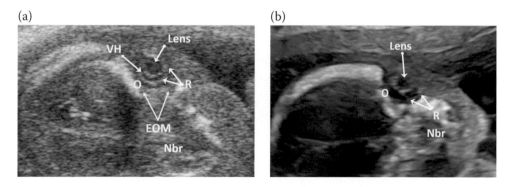

FIGURE 4.6 A: 15.5 dpc The mouse eye anatomy including orbit (O), lens of the eye, and nasal bridge (Nbr) are demarcated by this gestational age, but can be seen as early as 13.5 dpc. The lenses are seen as central circles that do not have an internal echogenicity. The extrinsic ocular muscles (EOM) and bones of the nasal bridge (Nbr) – which offer orientation to the midline of the face are seen. **B:** The human eye anatomy includes all analogous structures of the mouse at this midgestational time point. The structures of the orbit (O), lens of the eye (L) and nasal bridge (Nbr) are in the same anatomical orientation for each species. The extrinsic ocular muscles (EOM) are not as easily noted in the human fetus during ultrasound.

HUMAN

Imaging the spine and skin line in the sagittal plan offers the best views of intact skin as well as ossification of the vertebral body and the vertebral laminae. The vertebral column can be assessed in the coronal, axial, and longitudinal/sagittal planes. On ultrasound, the vertebrae will have three detectable ossification centers. These are the vertebral body anteriorly and two vertebral arches (or laminae) posteriorly. In the axial section, the three ossification centers are in a triangular arrangement.

MOUSE

Similar to the human, the mouse has cervical, thoracic, lumbar and sacral vertebrae within the spinal cord. Mice also have a caudal region which constitutes the tail. Analogous to the human, ultrasound is able to visualize the ossification of the vertebral body and the ossification centers of the vertebral lamina, in addition to the skin line, to aid in confirmation of continuous skin.

ANOMALIES

Neural tube defects (NTDs), including spina bifida are the most common of central nervous system malformations which are compatible with life. Spina bifida is heterogeneous and is thought to occur under the influence of both genetic and environmental factors; thus mouse models have proven to be a useful tool in identifying underlying genetic and environmental causes of neural tube defects (22), with over 250 mouse models with NTDs have been identified (23,24). See Figs. 4.7–4.12.

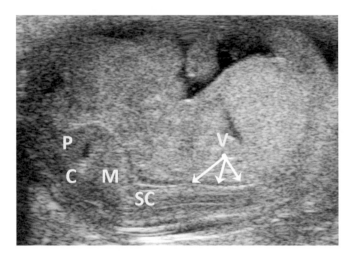

FIGURE 4.7 D13.5 – in the sagittal view, with the posterior fossa and the spinal cord are easily identified. In both the mouse and the human during fetal development, the fetal body is flexed anteriorly into the "fetal position", giving the entire vertebral column a single curve that is oriented in a concave shape anteriorly. The medulla oblongata (M), pons, spinal cord (SC) and vertebrae (V) are seen.

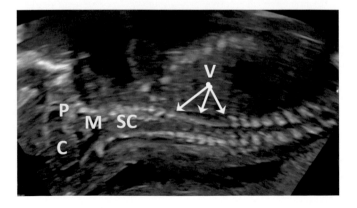

FIGURE 4.8 The human brain stem and spine at this mid gestational age are quite analogous to the mouse. Structures such as the medulla oblongata (M), pons (P), spinal cord (SC) and vertebrae (V) are seen in the same orientation and relative location compared to the mouse. Of note, the human fetal body is not as continuously flexed anteriorly as the mouse.

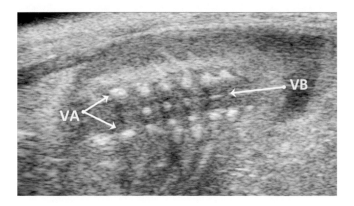

FIGURE 4.9 At 14.5 dpc, the most caudal region can be seen, with the vertebral processes apparent. As shown the paired vertebral arches (VA) ossification and the midline vertebral body (VB) ossification sites are seen easily in this coronal plane.

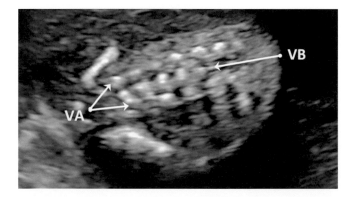

FIGURE 4.10 In the human at this gestational age, similar structures to the fetal mouse are appreciated. The midline vertebral and lateral vertebral arches are seen, and appear in a very similar manner to the murine fetus at this gestational age. The iliac crests are more easily visualized in the human fetus in this view compared to the mouse; this view is no able to be obtained in the fetal mouse at this gestational age.

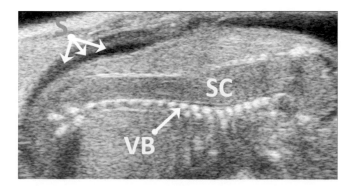

FIGURE 4.11 D15.5 spine – the long axis of the spine, including the spinal cord, cervical spine, vertebrae, and ribs, can be nicely imaged in the mouse. The sagittal view offers documentation of spinal development, and allow the identification of spinal anomalies or neural tube defects. Both the murine and human imaging allows for the spinal cord to be visualized from the middle to the caudal portion. The skin line (S) is also visible in the sagittal plane.

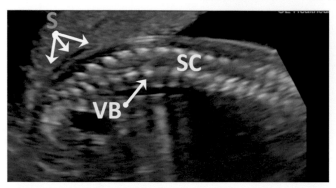

FIGURE 4.12 Similar to the mouse during mid-gestation, ultrasound of the human in the sagittal view allows the identification of spinal anomalies or neural tube defects. The spinal cord (SC) and vertebral bodies (VB) are both seen; this allows for comparison of spinal cord development. In cases of meningocele and myelomeningocele, the sac is best seen in these posterior longitudinal and posterior transaxial planes. The skin line (S) is also visible in the sagittal plane and should be imaged to evaluate for meningocele and myelomeningocele.

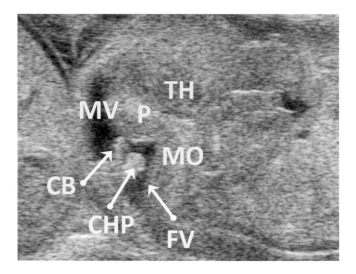

FIGURE 4.13 D13.5 – in this sagittal image, the lateral ventricle (LV), fourth ventricle (FV), mesencephalic ventricle (MV), and third ventricle (TV) are identified. The thalamus (TH), pons (P) and medulla oblongata (MO) serve as a landmark for these structures. The individual structures of the cerebellum (CB) and choroid plexus (CHP) best visualized in this sagittal view.

BRAIN

While the location and relative relationship of intracranial structures may vary between the mouse and human, numerous structures are presents and identifiable in both species. When comparing the two species, it is important to note that in the mouse, the changes that occur from late gestation 15 dpc through the first 10 days of postnatal neurodevelopment are equivalent to development of the human fetal brain during the third trimester of gestation (25,26). Thus, the development of fetal mouse structures seen during gestation are not as advanced as human structures detected prenatally.

HUMAN

The brain undergoes dynamic change and growth during the second trimester. From 11 weeks gestation, the choroid plexuses, seen as brightly echogenic structures, fill the large lateral ventricles

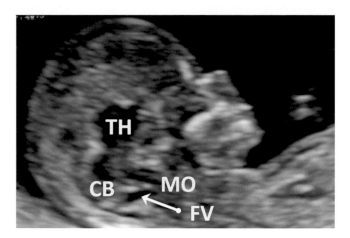

FIGURE 4.14 Sagittal – Very early in the second trimester, the sagittal, or profile images of the human fetus offer detection of similar structures as the mouse. In this view, similar to the mouse, structures such as the fourth ventricle (FV), cerebellum (CB) and the medulla oblongata (MO) are seen. The thalamus (TH) also serves as an important landmark.

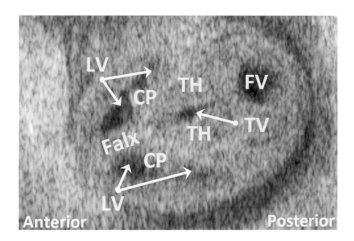

FIGURE 4.15 D13.5 – The transverse image of the brain allows for the right and left hemispheres to be imaged. These structures include the fourth ventricle (FV), third ventricle (TV), thalamus (TH) structures, midline falx cerebri (Falx), and lateral ventricles (LV) with the associated choroid plexus (CP). The chorioid plexus is less distinct in the mouse compared to the human, while the fourth ventricle is more distinct. The diameter of the lateral ventricle in the mouse at this gestational age is measured at 0.5 mm.

and early in the second trimester are the most prominent structures. The size of the lateral ventricles are reliably measured after 17 weeks (27). The first projections from the thalamus to cortex will begin to appear from 12 to 16 weeks gestation, and reliably measured via ultrasound from 20 weeks and onward (28). The cerebellum can be imaged from 19 to 20 weeks onward. In general, unless major structural anomalies are present, abnormalities are often not identified until after 20–22 weeks, as structures are not yet fully developed before this timeframe.

MOUSE

Rapid differentiation of the mouse brain occurs from 13.5 to 15.5 dpc, allowing ultrasound to reliably detect and measure such structures as the lateral ventricles, choroid plexus, thalamus, third

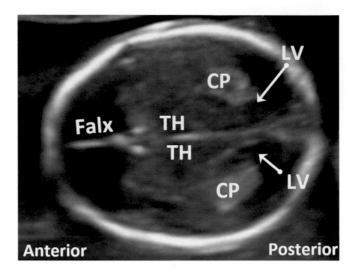

FIGURE 4.16 During the second trimester, the transverse axial planes in the human will reveal anatomy very similar to the mouse at this midgestational age. Analogous structures include the third ventricle (not seen in this image above, but which is flanked by the thalamus (TH) structures), midline falx cerebri (Falx), and lateral ventricles (LV) with the associated choroid plexus (CP). The average diameter of the lateral ventricle in the second trimester ranges from 6 to 7 mm [27], while the diameter in the mouse is 0.5 mm.

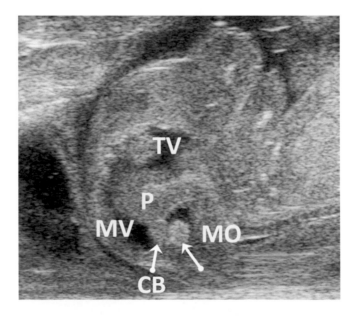

FIGURE 4.17 D14.5 Sagittal – sagittal images allow for the third ventricle (TV), mesencephalic ventricle (MV), pons (P), and the medulla oblongata (MO) to be determined. Even more apparent are the individual structures of the posterior structures of the cerebellum (CB) and choroid plexus (CP).

ventricle, fourth ventricle, cerebellum, pons, medulla oblongata, and falx cerebri. It is important to consider that the development of cerebellar foliation in the mouse occurs within the first two weeks after birth, during the post-natal life; subsequently, the hindbrain structures are not as well developed in the fetal mouse compared to the fetal human (29). The developing cerebellum is not easily visualized in the fetal mouse during gestation (30,31).

ANOMALIES

Central nervous system malformations are common abnormalities detected prenatally. Measurement of the lateral cerebral ventricles is attainable in mouse and human species, and can detect ranges of ventriculomegaly. To date, mouse models have provided important insights into the pathogenesis of numerous human anomalies, including congenital and neonatal hydrocephalus (32,33), ventriculomegaly (34,35), cephalocele (36), holoprosencephaly (37), and Dandy-Walker malformation (38). See Figs. 4.13–4.22.

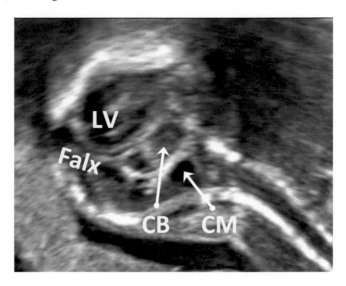

FIGURE 4.18 The structures of the cerebellum (CB), falx cerebri (Falx), posterior horn of the lateral ventricle (LV), and cisterna magna (CM) are seen in this view. The hindbrain of the mouse and posterior fossa in humans are quite different on ultrasound, compared to other more analogous structures. Most notably, the cerebellum is more distinct in the human, while the mouse has a more prominent pons on ultrasound.

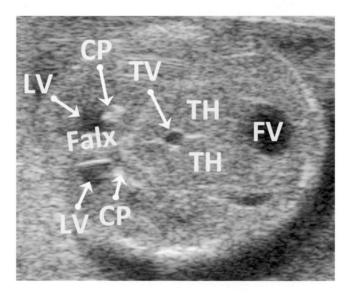

FIGURE 4.19 D14.5 – In both the mouse and the human, obtaining slightly different angles in cross-sections of brain structures in the transverse plane will result in different imaging opportunities for anatomy in the same plane. At 14.5 dpc, the following structures are still easily visualized: the large fourth ventricle (FV), third ventricle (TV) flanked by the thalamus (TH) structures, midline falx cerebri (Falx), and lateral ventricles (LV) with the associated choroid plexus (CP).

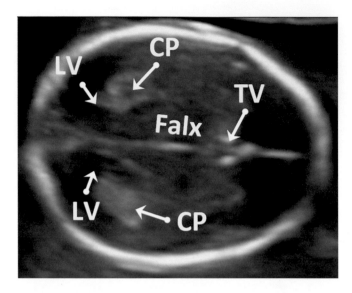

FIGURE 4.20 The midgestational brain anatomy in the human reveals similar structures to the mouse. Notably, the fourth ventricle is significantly less prominent in the human fetus, while the structures of the third ventricle (TV), thalamus (TH), midline falx cerebri (Falx), and lateral ventricles (LV) with the associated choroid plexus (CP) are easily identified in the mouse and human in different transverse planes of the brain.

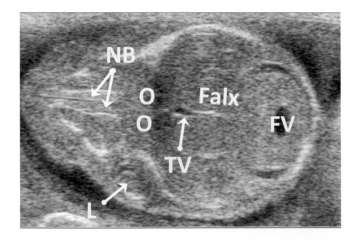

FIGURE 4.21 D15.5 – In both the mouse and the human, similar structures are still easily visualized: the large fourth ventricle (FV), and the third ventricle (TV) and midline falx cerebri structures. In the mouse, the olfactory bulbs (O) and nasal bones (NB) are easily visualized and more distinct than the human structures. The lens (L) can be seen in this cross section as well. The hindbrain structures such as the cerebellum and cisterna magna are still quite small and not detectable via ultrasound in the fetal mouse at this gestational age.

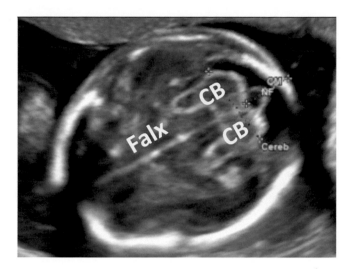

FIGURE 4.22 In midgestation in the human, the transaxial view can provide assessment of the posterior brain structures. In humans, the cerebellum (CB) shaped similar to a dumbbell, with symmetrical lobes. Measuring the trans-cerebellar diameter (Cereb) is the widest measurement across the cerebellum, perpendicular to the falx. Measurements of the cisterna magna (CM) and nuchal fold (NF), which are commonly obtained in the human, cannot be obtained in the fetal mouse via ultrasound.

REFERENCES

1. Bolon, B., *Pathology of the developing mouse: a systematic approach*. 2015, Boca Raton: CRC Press, Taylor & Francis Group. xvi, 430 pages.
2. Nyberg, D. A., Sickler, G. K., Hegge, F. N., Kramer, D. J. and Kropp, R. J., Fetal cleft-lip with and without cleft-palate – US classification and correlation with outcome. *Radiology*, 1995. 195(3): 677–684.
3. Jones, M. C., Prenatal diagnosis of cleft lip and palate: detection rates, accuracy of ultrasonography, associated anomalies, and strategies for counseling. *Cleft Palate Craniofac J*, 2002. 39(2): 169–173.
4. Stanier, P. and Moore, G. E., Genetics of cleft lip and palate: syndromic genes contribute to the incidence of non-syndromic clefts. *Hum Mol Genet*, 2004. 13 Spec No 1: R73–R81.
5. Tonni, G., Centini, G. and Rosignoli, L., Prenatal screening for fetal face and clefting in a prospective study on low-risk population: can 3- and 4-dimensional ultrasound enhance visualization and detection rate? *Oral Surg Oral Med Oral Pathol Oral Radiol Endod*, 2005. 100(4): 420–426.
6. Tonni, G., et al., Early detection of cleft lip by three-dimensional transvaginal ultrasound in niche mode in a fetus with trisomy 18 diagnosed by celocentesis. *Cleft Palate Craniofac J*, 2016. 53(6): 745–748.
7. Zajicek, M., et al., Sonographic assessment of fetal secondary palate between 12 and 16 weeks of gestation using three-dimensional ultrasound. *Prenat Diagn*, 2013. 33(13): 1256–1259.
8. Bush, J. O. and Jiang, R., Palatogenesis: morphogenetic and molecular mechanisms of secondary palate development. *Development*, 2012. 139(2): 231–243.
9. Gritli-Linde, A., Molecular control of secondary palate development. *Dev Biol*, 2007. 301(2): 309–326.
10. Christ, J. E. and Meininger, M. G., Ultrasound diagnosis of cleft lip and cleft palate before birth. *Plast Reconstr Surg*, 1981. 68(6): 854–859.
11. Gritli-Linde, A., The etiopathogenesis of cleft lip and cleft palate: usefulness and caveats of mouse models. *Curr Top Dev Biol*, 2008. 84: 37–138.
12. Ondeck, C. L., et al., Ultrasonographic prenatal imaging of fetal ocular and orbital abnormalities. *Surv Ophthalmol*, 2018. 63(6): 745–753.
13. Foster, F. S., et al., In vivo imaging of embryonic development in the mouse eye by ultrasound biomicroscopy. *Invest Ophthalmol Vis Sci*, 2003. 44(6): 2361–2366.
14. Dudas, M. and Kaartinen, V., Tgf-beta superfamily and mouse craniofacial development: interplay of morphogenetic proteins and receptor signaling controls normal formation of the face. *Curr Top Dev Biol*, 2005. 66: 65–133.

15. Cobourne, M. T., et al., Sonic hedgehog signalling inhibits palatogenesis and arrests tooth development in a mouse model of the nevoid basal cell carcinoma syndrome. *Dev Biol*, 2009. 331(1): 38–49.
16. Suzuki, A., et al., Molecular mechanisms of midfacial developmental defects. *Dev Dyn*, 2016. 245(3): 276–293.
17. Romain, M., et al., Prenatal ultrasound detection of congenital cataract in trisomy 21. *Prenat Diagn*, 1999. 19(8): 780–782.
18. Ghim, S., et al., Cataracts in transgenic mice caused by a human papillomavirus type 18 E7 oncogene driven by KRT1-14. *Exp Mol Pathol*, 2008. 85(2): 77–82.
19. Irum, B., et al., Mutation in LIM2 is responsible for autosomal recessive congenital cataracts. *PLoS One*, 2016. 11(11): p. e0162620.
20. Smith, R. S., Sundberg, J. P. and Linder, C. C., Mouse mutations as models for studying cataracts. *Pathobiology*, 1997. 65(3): 146–154.
21. Sadler, T. W., Embryology of neural tube development. *Am J Med Genet C Semin Med Genet*, 2005. 135C(1): 2–8.
22. Mohd-Zin, S. W., et al., Spina bifida: pathogenesis, mechanisms, and genes in mice and humans. *Scientifica (Cairo)*, 2017. 2017: 29. doi:10.1155/2017/5364827.
23. Copp, A. J. and Greene, N. D., Neural tube defects – disorders of neurulation and related embryonic processes. *Wiley Interdiscip Rev Dev Biol*, 2013. **2**(2): 213–227.
24. Harris, M. J. and Juriloff, D. M., An update to the list of mouse mutants with neural tube closure defects and advances toward a complete genetic perspective of neural tube closure. *Birth Defects Res A Clin Mol Teratol*, 2010. 88(8): 653–669.
25. Clancy, B., et al., Extrapolating brain development from experimental species to humans. *Neurotoxicology*, 2007. 28(5): 931–937.
26. Workman, A. D., et al., Modeling transformations of neurodevelopmental sequences across mammalian species. *J Neurosci*, 2013. 33(17): 7368–7383.
27. Salomon, L. J., Bernard, J. P. and Ville, Y., Reference ranges for fetal ventricular width: a non-normal approach. *Ultrasound Obstet Gynecol*, 2007. 30(1): 61–66.
28. Sotiriadis, A., et al., Thalamic volume measurement in normal fetuses using three-dimensional sonography. *J Clin Ultrasound*, 2012. 40(4): 207–213.
29. Chizhikov, V. and Millen, K. J., Development and malformations of the cerebellum in mice. *Mol Genet Metab*, 2003. 80(1–2): 54–65.
30. Blaess, S., Corrales, J. D. and Joyner, A. L., Sonic hedgehog regulates Gli activator and repressor functions with spatial and temporal precision in the mid/hindbrain region. *Development*, 2006. 133(9): 1799–1809.
31. Sudarov, A. and A. L. Joyner, Cerebellum morphogenesis: the foliation pattern is orchestrated by multicellular anchoring centers. *Neural Dev*, 2007. 2: 26.
32. Konishi, S., et al., Pathological characteristics of Ccdc85c knockout rats: a rat model of genetic hydrocephalus. *Exp Anim*, 2019. 69: 26–33.
33. McAllister, J. P. 2nd, Pathophysiology of congenital and neonatal hydrocephalus. *Semin Fetal Neonatal Med*, 2012. 17(5): 285–294.
34. McKechnie, L., Vasudevan, C. and Levene, M., Neonatal outcome of congenital ventriculomegaly. *Semin Fetal Neonatal Med*, 2012. 17(5): 301–307.
35. Mero, I. L., et al., Homozygous KIDINS220 loss-of-function variants in fetuses with cerebral ventriculomegaly and limb contractures. *Hum Mol Genet*, 2017. 26(19): 3792–3796.
36. Fong, K. S., et al., Midline craniofacial malformations with a lipomatous cephalocele are associated with insufficient closure of the neural tube in the tuft mouse. *Birth Defects Res A Clin Mol Teratol*, 2014. 100(8): 598–607.
37. Grinblat, Y. and Lipinski, R. J., A forebrain undivided: unleashing model organisms to solve the mysteries of holoprosencephaly. *Dev Dyn*, 2019. 248(8): 626–633.
38. Blank, M. C., et al., Multiple developmental programs are altered by loss of Zic1 and Zic4 to cause Dandy-Walker malformation cerebellar pathogenesis. *Development*, 2011. 138(6): 1207–1216.

5 Late-Gestation and Third Trimester

Mouse D16.5–18.5; Human 28–40 Weeks

As discussed previously, human and mouse fetal development timelines differ in the later trimesters. For mice, the third or "last" trimester is considered to include the development after 15.5 dpc and up until the 10th post-natal day after birth. Thus, while human trimesters cease at birth, the final developmental stages of the mouse will include developments that occur after birth (1). This publication does not include ultrasound during the postnatal period of the mouse.

KIDNEYS

The urinary system, comprised of the kidneys, ureters, bladder and urethra are responsible for the production and release of urine (2). Mammalian renal development which includes the differentiation from pronephros, mesonephros, and metanephros; the metanephros persists as the definitive adult kidney, and has a branched collecting duct system and many nephrons (3,4).

HUMAN

The human kidney is functional around 11 weeks of gestation, which corresponds to embryonic stages 15.5–16.5 dpc in mice. A detailed evaluation of human fetal kidney and renal pelvis by ultrasound has been documented as early as 12 weeks, although the fetal kidney is most reliably visualized as the second trimester progresses (2,5). The kidneys are seen as paired hypoechoic structures on either side of the fetal spine. In the third trimester, the kidneys are easily identified by imaging the dorsolumbar spine and scanning on either side in both the sagittal and transverse axial sections (6).

MOUSE

In the mouse, the metanephros development is initiated at 10.5 dpc; however the mouse kidneys are not able to be reliably visualized by ultrasound until 15.5 dpc, when the renal pelvis can be both identified and measured at this time. Ultrasound has been used previously to assess mouse fetal renal development, and, as shown here, the earliest detection is 15.5 dpc, when the kidney starts to produce urine, allowing the renal pelvis to be seen (7).

ANOMALIES

Antenatal hydronephrosis and vesicoureteral reflux (VUR) have been successfully modeled in mice to investigate pathophysiology (8), along with murine ultrasound techniques (7). As the kidneys start producing urine at 15.5 dpc, pathologies in the mouse are identified from 16.5–18.5 dpc (7,9). Mouse renal ultrasound imaging can measure diagnose the degree of pelviectasis or hydronephrosis in the anteroposterior measurement in the same manner as the human fetus (10). See Figs. 5.1–5.2.

(a)   (b)

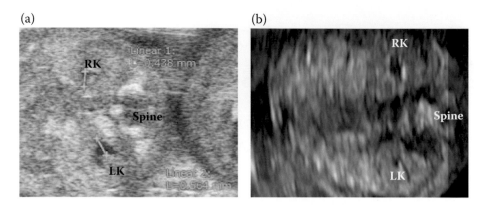

FIGURE 5.1 A: 16.5 dpc – The spine (Spine) is in the midline posterior position, flanked by the two kidneys (K). The renal pelvis (Rp) is still seen as a dark, anechoic areas in the central portion of the kidney, and the degree of pelviectasis or hydronephrosis can be quantified. The typical renal pelvis measures approximately between 0.4 mm and 0.5 mm in diameter. **B:** Ultrasound imaging of the human renal system can also measure the degree of pelviectasis or hydronephrosis in the anteroposterior measurement. The images are taken in the same plane, with the two kidneys lateral to the fetal spine (S). As in the mouse, the renal pelvis is seen as a dark, anechoic areas in the central portion of the kidney.

(a)   (b)

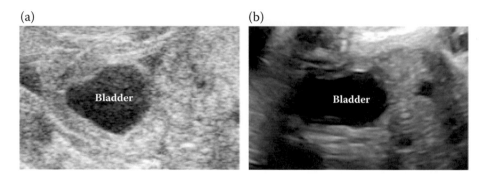

FIGURE 5.2 A: 17.5 dpc – The dimensions of a typical mouse fetal bladder in later gestation will range from 1.5 to 2.5 mm in diameter. In the example image shown above, the dimensions are 1.7 mm × 2.2 mm, representing a normal fetal bladder size. **B:** In the third trimester, the human fetal bladder is visualized in the same manner as the mouse fetal bladder; it will appear as a circular or oval-shaped anechoic (black) area in the anterior region of the fetal pelvis. The similarities in both the shape and location of mouse and human fetal bladder views is appreciable in these comparison images.

HEART

The formation of the heart is very similar in the mouse and the human fetus. The structures of the heart are developed by 14.5 dpc, and will continue to grow in size in the following gestational days. Embryologically, the mouse cardiac structures at 14.5 dpc are similar to human fetal cardiac structures at 7 weeks to 8 weeks of gestation. These very similar comparisons of mouse and human cardiac development permit the use of mouse cardiac morphogenesis as an excellent model for human pathophysiology of the cardiovascular system (11).

HUMAN

In the third trimester, cardiac anatomy such as the four-chamber view (size and shape of ventricles and atria), valves, left and right ventricular outflow tracts, aortic and ductal arch, superior and inferior vena cava views are visualized. This is most often evaluated via a specialized fetal echocardiogram (12). Due to the marked size difference between the mouse and human fetal heart, more structures are easily identified in the human fetus; to date no specialized mouse "fetal echocardiogram" has been developed, likely due to the inability to achieve a more targeted ultrasound than the current general mouse fetal ultrasound offers.

MOUSE

Ultrasound has been successfully used to assess the flow and distribution in the mouse fetal circulation in utero (13) and with the additional of color Doppler, anatomy can be further characterized. Measurements of systolic and diastolic cardiac function, as well as distribution of blood flow within the developing fetal body are thus detectable (14). Within the heart, chamber wall thickness, lumen dimensions in both systole and diastole can help detect hypertrophy of the ventricular myocardium (15).

ANOMALIES

It is important to recognize that the mouse fetal circulatory system is quite similar to humans in the major vessels and orientations, but differs in that there is are bilateral superior vena cavae and only a single umbilical artery (16). The use of genetically engineered mouse models have been successfully used to explore the role of genes in normal and abnormal cardiovascular development (17–19). Comparison between mouse and fetal cardiovascular development can be monitored and compared with non-invasive ultrasound monitoring (19–21). A variety of congenital cardiac defects have been modeled in mice, including heterotaxy with single ventricle (22), defects in left-right symmetry (23). See Figs. 5.3–5.6.

EYE AND ORBIT

The eye forms originates from several cell types, including ectoderm, neural crest cells, and mesenchyme. The neural tube ectoderm will give rise to the retina, the iris, optic nerve, and some of the vitreous humor, while the surface ectoderm will give rise to the lens, and eyelids. The remaining ocular structures originate from mesenchyme. Both mouse and human ocular anatomy are very similar under ultrasound surveillance during fetal development; similar structures are seen in each.

HUMAN

Eye formation begins at approximately three weeks into embryonic development and continues through the tenth week. However, ocular structures such as the vitreous humor, retina, and lens are

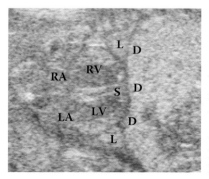

FIGURE 5.3   15.5 dpc – The ventricles of the heart can be seen in both the cardiac diastole and systole. In the image above, the heart is in diastole with both the right (RV) and left ventricles (LV), right atrium (RA) and left atrium (LA) labeled, as well as the ventricular septum (S). The intracardiac blood is seen as a darker shade of grey, while the cardiac myometrium (wall of the ventricles) appear as a lighter grey. Structures of the diaphragm (D) and the right and left lungs (L) can been identified.

(a)   (b)

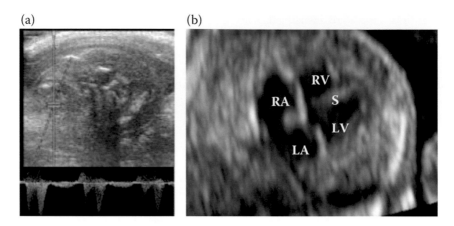

FIGURE 5.4 A: The pulse wave Doppler (above) allows for the fetal heart to be audibly detected and the fetal heart rate to be quantified. **B:** In the human, the ventricles appear very similar to the mouse; the right (RV) and left ventricles (LV) are prominent with the intact septal wall dividing.

(a)   (b)

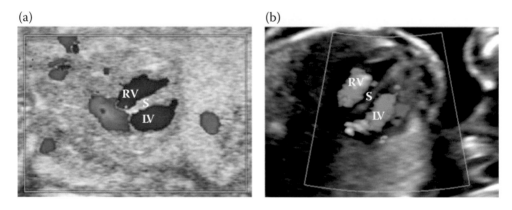

FIGURE 5.5 A: D16.5 – The black coloring represents the ventricular blood flow in the right (RV) and left (LV) ventricles; as can be easily seen, there separating septum (S) between each ventricular chamber, indicating the absence of a ventricular septal wall defect. **B:** In the human fetus at a similar gestational age, color doppler is also used to identify similar blood flow patterns among the cardiac chambers. The blood flow in each ventricular chamber is seen, with the septum dividing, thus demonstrating the absence of a ventricular wall defect.

more reliably monitored via ultrasound in the second and third trimesters (24). It should also be noted that the eyelids open in the mouse approximately two weeks after birth, while in humans, they open at around 28 weeks of gestation.

MOUSE

Similar to human fetal imaging, ocular structures such as the vitreous and lens are reliably seen via ultrasound in late gestation (25). In CD-1 mice, the lens grows approximately 68 μm a day, and the globe grows at 122 μm a day (26). As has been reported previously, both the lid and iris are challenging to visualize with ultrasound, due to similar echogenicity with surrounding tissue. The structures that are more reliably seen include the lens, vitreous humor, retina, and posterior retinal space (26).

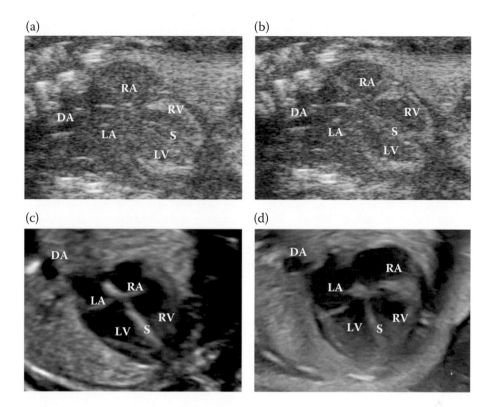

FIGURE 5.6 AB: D18.5 – During the later gestational ages, the cardiac anatomy is more clearly defined. Both the right (RV) and left ventricles (LV) are easily seen, positioned caudal to the right (RA) and left (LA) atria. Again, the intracardiac blood is seen as a darker shade of grey, while the cardiac myometrium is a lighter grey. For reference, the thickness of the ventricular septum is approximately 0.6 mm at this gestational age. In the above examples, the heart is 3.7 mm × 3.0 mm in size. 6CD During later gestational ages in the human, the same four chamber view is easily demarcated. Both the right (RV) and left ventricles (LV) and right (RA) and left (LA) atria as can be appreciated. Structures such as the ventricular septum (S) and the descending aorta (DA) are analogous to the mouse. The four chambers structure of the fetal human heart and murine fetal hard are very similar.

Anomalies

Abnormalities in ocular growth have been associated with abnormal cerebral development and congenital syndromes that present with features of microphthalmos and anophthalmos (24). Additionally, transgenic mouse models have produced anomalies seen in humans, including glaucoma, retinal and macular degeneration, cataracts, retinoblastoma, and intraocular tumors, as reviewed (26). See Figs. 5.7–5.8.

LIMBS, HANDS, FEET AND PAWS

The development of upper and lower limbs, paws in mice and hands/feet in humans continues through the third trimester. While in each species anomalies have most likely occurred before these later gestational dates, the increased size allows for more clear delineation of the long bone growth and development of digits. In each of these skeletal structures, the ossified areas are more visible under ultrasound guidance, and are thus even more readily quantified (27).

(a)   (b)

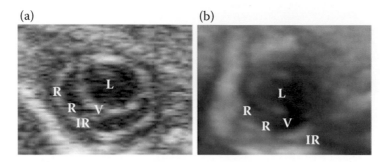

FIGURE 5.7 A: Mouse 18.5 – The vitreous humor (V), retina (R), and lens (L), and intraretinal space (IR) are reliably seen. The thickness of the retina is 0.1 mm (100 µm) and the diameter of the lens at this gestational age is approximately 0.7–0.8 mm. **B:** The human eye in the third trimester is developed enough to visualize the vitreous humor (V), retina (R), and lens (L), and intraretinal space (IR). These structures appear quite similar to the anatomy of the fetal mouse. Of note, the human fetal eyelids are open in utero at this time, while the mouse fetal eyelids are closed in utero and remain closed at the time of birth.

(a)   (b)

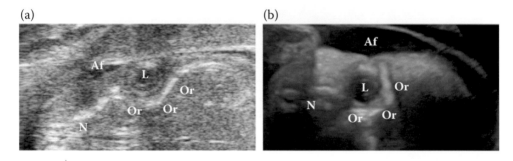

FIGURE 5.8 A: Mouse 17.5 – The lens of the eye (L), bones of the orbit (Or) and nasal bones (N) can all be obtained in this coronal plane view. There is often a pocket of amniotic fluid (Af) near the facial structures, which can be appreciated in both humans and mice. **B:** Human – in the same coronal plane view, structures of the human lens of the eye (L), bones of the orbit (Or) and nasal bones (N) can all be obtained in this coronal plane view. The pocket of amniotic fluid (Af) is seen as a hypoechoic black pocket of fluid near the facial structures, similar to that seen in the mouse.

HUMAN

The formation of the hands, feet, fingers and toes can be initially determined in the second trimester, however are better characterized in the third trimester, as the structures increase in size (28) via 2D and 3D ultrasound (29,30). Measurements of long bones in the human fetal period via ultrasound have been helpful to detect anomalies and predict postnatal abnormalities (31).

MOUSE

The long bones of the limb continue to grow in the axial direction during late gestation, with structures such as the clavicle, humerus, radius and ulna continue to grow and become more apparent by ultrasound due to continued ossification. In the mouse, during embryonic days 9.5–12.5 dpc the progenitors that will give rise to the future skeletal elements continue to grow and are patterned. As the long bones are more easily measured in later gestation, anomalies that have occurred earlier in development may now be more reliably detected (27).

ANOMALIES

Abnormalities in the hand or digit morphology can be detected, including clenched hand, club-hand, thumb anomalies, abnormal size or number. Mouse models have been routinely used to identify genetic and environmental contributions to limb and digit defects (32,33), as well as investigate molecular contributions to a wide range of skeletal dyplasias that are modeled in mice (34). The length of the long bones such as femur and humerus can help determine risk for fetal aneuploidy or skeletal dysplasia (35). See Figs. 5.9–5.14.

(a) (b)

(c) (d)

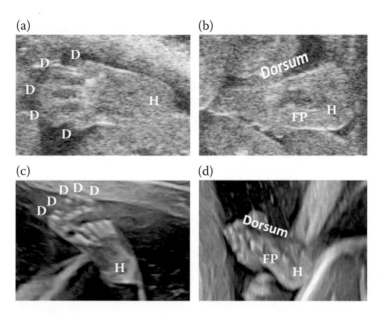

FIGURE 5.9 AB: Mouse 16.5 – The mouse paw is identified as a "foot print" that reveals the number, position, and general morphology of the digits (D). As in the human, the mouse has five digits. However, in the mouse, the three digits in the center are similar in length and the two flanking digits are significantly shorter. In the image on the right at 17.5 dpc, the sagittal or "side view" of the murine hind paw demonstrates the heel (H), foot pad (FP), and dorsum structures. 9 CD Human – Similar to the mouse, the digits (D) and heel are easily identified. The image on the right is analogous to the sagittal or "side view" of the murine hind paw and demonstrates the human heel (H), foot pad (FP), and top of the foot (Dorsum).

(a) (b)

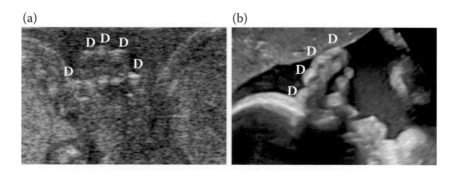

FIGURE 5.10 A: Mouse 17.5 dpc – The five digits of the mouse forepaw (analogous to the human hand) is seen, allowing for both the number and relative location of each digit to be quantified. Fetal crowding can often limit the evaluation of each hand. **B:** It is important to note that the human fetal hand is often curled "closed", while the mouse fetal forepaw/hand is often in a flat or "open" position. Consequently, in the human, the four digits (D) are often seen in one plane, without the thumb.

(a)   (b)

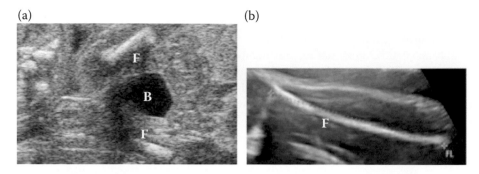

FIGURE 5.11 A: Mouse D18.5 – The femur at this gestational age is 1.2 mm in length and 0.25–0.3 mm in diameter. Both femurs (F) are visible in this view, however the femur at the top of the image is the most elongated to provide an accurate measurement. The fetal bladder (B) is seen between the femurs. Even as early as 16.5 dpc the femur is obtained in the transverse view of the fetus, measuring approximately 0.9 mm in length and 0.27 mm in diameter. At 17.5 dpc, it measures 1.1 mm in length and 0.4 mm in diameter. **B:** In the third trimester, the ossified femur is easily measured as a linear white line within the lower limb. Compared to the mouse, the femur bone is more elongated, however still appears in the analogous anatomical location. For comparison, the femur length in this image at 35 weeks gestation is 6.88 cm, while the femur length of the fetal mouse at 18.5 dpc is approximately 0.122 cm.

(a)   (b)

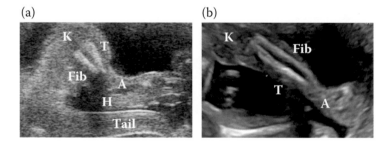

FIGURE 5.12 A: Mouse 16.5 – the tibia (T) and fibula (Fib) long bones are seen as two elongated hyperchoic areas in the lower portion of the hind limb, between the knee (K) and the ankle (A). In this image, the tibia measures 1.26 mm in length and fibula measures 1.09 mm. Both are similar in diameter between 0.2 and 0.25 mm at this gestational age. The heel (H) and tail are also seen. **B:** The long bones of the lower leg of the human are assessed in a similar manner to the mouse. The tibia (T) and fibula (Fib) long bones should be seen in each leg and are of approximate equal length. A sagittal side on image of each leg will demonstrate the ankle to be correctly orientated. The leg should not be visible in same plane as the sole of the foot.

FACE AND SNOUT

During early craniofacial development, the embryos of mice and humans look similar. This intricate process of craniofacial formation occurs early in gestation, however the detection and magnitude of such anomalies more often occurs in the later gestation. It is important to recognize that successful imaging of the human and mouse facial features occurs when there is a small pocket of amniotic fluid in front of the face, to allow for delicate facial structures to be accessed.

HUMAN

Continued growth of the fetus allows for continued characterization of the type and severity of such defects though ultrasonography. In the human, standard 2D ultrasound can detect possible

(a) (b)

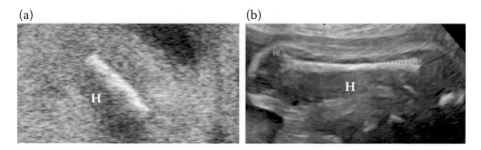

FIGURE 5.13 A: Mouse 17.5 – the humerus (H) is easily seen as a linear hyperechoic bone in the upper forelimb, extending from the shoulder. It is simple to identify as a linear hyperechoic bone in the upper forelimb, extending from the shoulder. At this gestational age, the humerus is 1.85 mm, 0.2–0.25 mm in width. 13B The human long bones have greater length compared to width, compared to the analogous bone in the mouse. In this image, the humerus measures 4.8 cm; by comparison, the mouse humerus measures 0.17–0.18 cm at this same gestational age.

(a) (b)

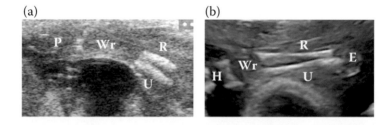

FIGURE 5.14 A: Mouse 16.5 dpc – in the lower portion of the right forelimb, the right ulna (U) and radius (R) bones are seen in this plane. In this image, the radius is 1.78 mm in length; the ulna measures 1.4 mm. The location of the elbow (E), wrist (Wr) and the forepaw (P) are labeled. **B:** In the human, the relative position and visualization of the radius (R) and ulna (U) are very similar to the mouse. The human elbow (E), wrist (Wr) and the hand (H) are all easily obtained in the analogous view.

cleft lip in both the coronal and axial planes, with the anterior coronal plane providing optimal views (36). Certain defects such as lateral clefts are most reliably detected with 3D ultrasound in particular (37).

MOUSE

Mouse pathogenesis starts at 11.5 dpc, with the formation of palatal shelves extending from the maxillae; between day 12.5 and 13.5 dpc, these shelves protrude downwards, on both sides of the tongue. Complete fusion of the palatal shelves occurs on day 14.5 dpc (38). Thus, ultrasounds of fetal facial features shown in these later gestational ages demonstrate any anomalies that have already been established in the fetus. However, these anomalies are more easily seen and detected at these later gestational ages, making ultrasound at this time quite useful.

ANOMALIES

Both species share genes that are involved in orofacial clefting and mouse models have been widely used to understand the development of facial defects (39). Multiple candidate single gene mutations in mice have also been implicated (40). These factors make murine studies of facial anomalies particularly useful, with prenatal ultrasound techniques valuable to understand the fetal development of such anomalies. See Fig. 5.15.

SPINE AND TAIL

The fetal central nervous system undergoes significant changes during the entire gestation. Sonography can identify the bright, echogenic ossification centers of the vertebrae, which are located with one in the center (medial) as well two laterally. While many defects occur before the end of gestation, the increased size of the fetus can allow for more accurate imaging of these structures, especially in the fetal mouse.

HUMAN

The human spine is quite amenable to characterization via ultrasound. Because of the length of the spinal column and position of the fetus, multiple images and planes are necessary to assess the complete length (41). Ultrasound performed at midgestation and late gestation is preferable for detecting anomalies, such as anencephaly and spina bifida (42). Sagittal views can detect defects in the spinal column or skin, while a coronal plane can detect the placement and lateral spacing of ossified spinal segments or enlargement of the spinal canal (43).

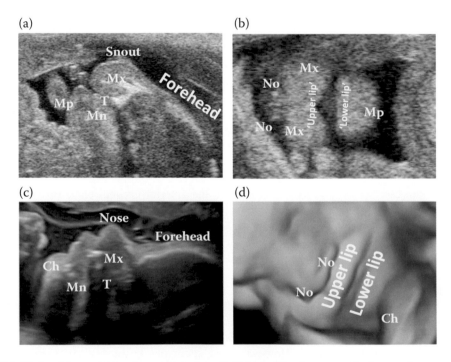

FIGURE 5.15 A: Mouse 16.5 – the sagittal plane (left) in profile; the mouse fetal snout is recognized and the maxillary bones are echogenic. In this sagittal view the mandible (Mn), maxilla (Mx), maxillary prominence (Mp; analogous to the human chin) and tongue (T) are seen. **B:** The frontal/coronal plane, the maxillary and mandibular prominences (somewhat analogous to the upper and lower lips/chin) are strikingly similar to the commonly obtained view of human nose, mouth, lips, and chin. The nostrils (No) of the mouse fetus are seen at the tip of the frontonasal process. 15C The human nose (analogous to snout), mandible (Mn), maxilla (Mx), chin (analogous to maxillary prominence) chin) and tongue (T) are all in the same orientation. **D:** 3D imaging allows excellent images of the front of the face. This can demonstrate two nostrils (No), intact upper and lower lips, and chin (Ch).

MOUSE

By this stage of embryonic development, the appearance of the spine is very similar to the adult. The regional differences between the cervical, thoracic, sacral and caudal (tail) portions are apparent due to their different characteristics (44). On ultrasound, the thoracic portions are identified as being associated with the ribs and rib cage and the sacral region located between the bones of the pelvis (ilium, ischium and pubis) (45). The caudal portion of the spinal cord is contained entirely within the tail of the mouse.

ANOMALIES

Multiple transgenic and mutant mouse models have been identified with these anomalies including open spina bifida, exencephaly, anencephaly and brain herniation (46), while ultrasounds of the human fetus have long allowed for prenatal diagnosis of these defects, with recent advances in in utero correction of anomalies, prior to birth (47). Consequently, applying ultrasound techniques to mice will allow for continued mouse models of diagnosis and intervention of these defects in utero. See Figs. 5.16–5.18.

BRAIN/CNS

The ability to measure the growth of the brain's fluid-filled spaces relative to the surrounding brain tissue can provide critical information to clinicians caring for developing fetuses. In later gestation, the specific brain structures are more easily characterized by ultrasound, especially in the human. In the mouse, the clarity and growth of individual brain structures are less pronounced, due to difficulties with fetal crowding and shadowing.

HUMAN

The typical axial ultrasound views of the posterior fossa are often used for routine scanning for fetal anomalies, with additional imaging possible using three-dimensional ultrasound techniques (48). The lateral ventricle volume slowly decreases during the second trimester and then will increase more rapidly in later gestation, from 24 to 35 weeks; of note, in the mouse the lumen of the lateral ventricles will decrease in size during later gestation.

(a)

(b)

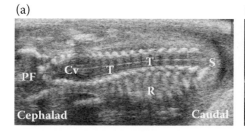
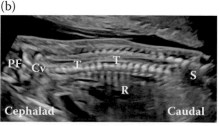

FIGURE 5.16 A: Mouse D16.5–17.5 – The posterior fossa (PF), cervical (Cv), thoracic (T), and sacral (S) spine are shown from an anterior-posterior view. The vertical echogenic lines representing ribs (R) of the thoracic region are seen flanking the thoracic vertebrae. Cephalad and caudal orientation labels are provided. **B:** Human – the same anterior-posterior view provides similar structures: posterior fossa (PF), cervical spinal column (Cv), thoracic (T), and sacral (S) spine are shown. As in the mouse, the vertical echogenic lines representing ribs (R) of the thoracic region are seen flanking the thoracic vertebrae.

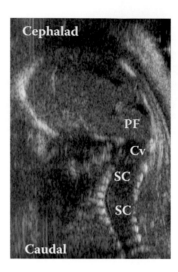

FIGURE 5.17 Mouse D18.5 –The sagittal view demonstrates the posterior fossa (PF), cervical spinal column (Cv), and spinal cord (SC).

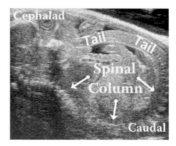

FIGURE 5.18 Mouse 18.5 – while there exists no human correlate to the elongated mouse tail, images of the typical size, location, and shape of mouse fetal tail are included. The sagittal plane demonstrates the overall morphology of the entire spinal column, in addition to the location of the tail which is consistently seen curling under the ventral side of the fetus, terminating near the face and the chest wall.

MOUSE

The intracranial structures are more difficult to delineate in the mouse fetus at this gestational age, as the cerebral cortex becomes increasingly laminated. The ventricular system becomes less prominent as cellular proliferation and differentiation occurs, particularly in the forebrain. This results in the lumen of the lateral ventricles to shrink in size and become less visible on ultrasound. Of note, significant maturation and growth of brain structures continue to occur after birth of the mouse pup.

ANOMALIES

Anomalies such as Dandy-Walker malformation, mega cisterna magna and other posterior fossa pathologies can be imaged in both mice and humans prenatally. Transgenic mouse models have been used to investigate causes of such anomalies as complex posterior fossa defects (including Dandy-Walker malformation) (49) as well as hydrocephalus due to a genetic mutations (50). Thus, the application of prenatal mouse ultrasound for emerging mouse models will serve as an excellent correlative monitoring system for the diagnosis and possible prenatal interventions. See Figs. 5.19–5.20.

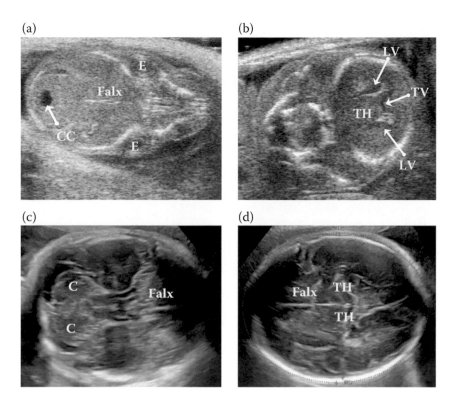

FIGURE 5.19 A: Mouse D17.5   The coronal image reveals the continued development of brain structures, including the central canal (CC), the falx cerebri, and eye (E). **B:** The frontal image plane image allows for the thalamus (TH), third ventricle (TV) and the lateral ventricle (LV) to be visualized. The size and dilation of the ventricles is critical in evaluating proper brain development. **C** In the later gestation in humans, the posterior structures of the brain are visualized, with each hemisphere of the cerebellum (C)labeled. The midline demarcated by the falx cerebri. 19D The human thalami (TH) are visualized as a central structure in each lobe. This provides orientation for imaging of other developing nearby structures.

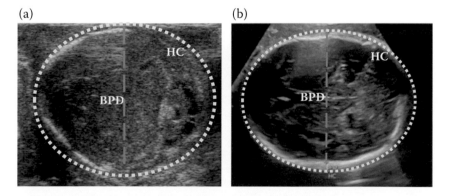

FIGURE 5.20 A: Mouse D17.5 – In a cross-sectional plane, the biparietal diameter (BPD, grey line) is obtained by measuring the distance from the other edge of the cranium on one side to the inner edge of the cranium on the opposite side. The head circumference (HC, white oval) is measured by the outer edge of the skull. The BPD in this image measures 5.9 mm and HC is 23.9 mm. **B:** Human third trimester – similar to the mouse, the biparietal diameter (BPD, grey line) and head circumference (HC, white oval) are readily obtained via ultrasound. The landmarks and measuring techniques are analogous in each species.

REFERENCES

1. Bolon, B., Pathology of the developing mouse: a systematic approach. 2015, Boca Raton: CRC Press, Taylor & Francis Group. xvi, 430 pages.

2. Ryan, D., et al., Development of the human fetal kidney from mid to late gestation in male and female infants. *EBioMedicine*, 2018. 27: 275–283.

3. Upadhyay, K. K. and Silverstein, D. M., Renal development: a complex process dependent on inductive interaction. *Curr Pediatr Rev*, 2014. 10(2): 107–114.

4. Bard, J. B., Growth and death in the developing mammalian kidney: signals, receptors and conversations. *Bioessays*, 2002. 24(1): 72–82.

5. Rosati, P. and Guariglia, L., Transvaginal sonographic assessment of the fetal urinary tract in early pregnancy. *Ultrasound Obstet Gynecol*, 1996. 7(2): 95–100.

6. Richmond, S. and Atkins, J., A population-based study of the prenatal diagnosis of congenital malformation over 16 years. *BJOG*, 2005. 112(10): 1349–1357.

7. Wang, H., Li, Q., Liu, J., Mendelsohn, C., Salant, D. J. and Lu, W., Noninvasive assessment of antenatal hydronephrosis in mice reveals a critical role for Robo2 in maintaining anti-reflux mechanism. *PLoS One*, 2011. 6(9): e24763.

8. Little, M. H., Kumar, S. V. and Forbes, T., Recapitulating kidney development: progress and challenges. *Semin Cell Dev Biol*, 2019. 91: 153–168.

9. Sherer, D. M., et al., Prenatal sonographic diagnosis of unilateral fetal renal agenesis. *J Clin Ultrasound*, 1990. 18(8): 648–652.

10. Dremsek, P. A., et al., Renal pyelectasis in fetuses and neonates: diagnostic value of renal pelvis diameter in pre- and postnatal sonographic screening. *AJR Am J Roentgenol*, 1997. 168(4): 1017–1019.

11. Krishnan, A., et al., A detailed comparison of mouse and human cardiac development. *Pediatr Res*, 2014. 76(6): 500–507.

12. Zhang, Y. F., et al., Diagnostic value of fetal echocardiography for congenital heart disease: a systematic review and meta-analysis. *Medicine (Baltimore)*, 2015. 94(42): e1759.

13. Zhou, Y. Q., et al., Assessment of flow distribution in the mouse fetal circulation at late gestation by high-frequency Doppler ultrasound. *Physiol Genomics*, 2014. 46(16): 602–614.

14. Liu, X., et al., Interrogating congenital heart defects with noninvasive fetal echocardiography in a mouse forward genetic screen. *Circ Cardiovasc Imaging*, 2014. 7(1): 31–42.

15. Maciver, R. D. and Ozolins, T. R. S., The application of high-resolution ultrasound for assessment of cardiac structure and function associated with developmental toxicity. *Methods Mol Biol*, 2019. 1965: 405–420.

16. Prsa, M., et al., Reference ranges of blood flow in the major vessels of the normal human fetal circulation at term by phase-contrast magnetic resonance imaging. *Circ Cardiovasc Imaging*, 2014. 7(4): 663–670.

17. Chin, A. J., Saint-Jeannet, J. P. and Lo, C. W., How insights from cardiovascular developmental biology have impacted the care of infants and children with congenital heart disease. *Mech Dev*, 2012. 129(5–8): 75–97.

18. Doetschman, T. and Azhar, M., Cardiac-specific inducible and conditional gene targeting in mice. *Circ Res*, 2012. 110(11): 1498–1512.

19. Phoon, C. K., et al., Embryonic heart failure in NFATc1-/- mice: novel mechanistic insights from in utero ultrasound biomicroscopy. *Circ Res*, 2004. 95(1): 92–99.

20. Phoon, C. K. and Turnbull, D. H., Ultrasound biomicroscopy-Doppler in mouse cardiovascular development. *Physiol Genomics*, 2003. 14(1): 3–15.

21. Liu, X., et al., Phenotyping cardiac and structural birth defects in fetal and newborn mice. *Birth Defects Res*, 2017. 109(10): 778–790.

22. Aune, C. N., et al., Mouse model of heterotaxy with single ventricle spectrum of cardiac anomalies. *Pediatr Res*, 2008. 63(1): 9–14.

23. Purandare, S. M., et al., A complex syndrome of left-right axis, central nervous system and axial skeleton defects in Zic3 mutant mice. *Development*, 2002. 129(9): 2293–2302.

24. Achiron, R., et al., The development of the fetal eye: in utero ultrasonographic measurements of the vitreous and lens. *Prenat Diagn*, 1995. 15(2): 155–160.

25. Turnbull, D. H., In utero ultrasound backscatter microscopy of early stage mouse embryos. *Comput Med Imaging Graph*, 1999. 23(1): 25–31.

26. Foster, F. S., et al., In vivo imaging of embryonic development in the mouse eye by ultrasound biomicroscopy. *Invest Ophthalmol Vis Sci*, 2003. 44(6): 2361–2366.

27. Zuniga, A., Next generation limb development and evolution: old questions, new perspectives. *Development*, 2015. 142(22): 3810–3820.

28. Stoll, C., et al., Evaluation of the prenatal diagnosis of limb reduction deficiencies. EUROSCAN Study Group. *Prenat Diagn*, 2000. 20(10): 811–818.

29. Gilboa, Y., et al., Prenatal diagnosis of fetal adducted thumbs. *J Matern Fetal Neonatal Med*, 2018. 31(10): 1285–1289.

30. Muscatello, A., et al., Correlation between 3D ultrasound appearance and postnatal findings in bilateral malformations of the fetal hands. *Fetal Diagn Ther*, 2012. 31(2): 138–140.

31. Pazzaglia, U. E., et al., Long bone human anlage longitudinal and circumferential growth in the fetal period and comparison with the growth plate cartilage of the postnatal age. *Microsc Res Tech*, 2019. 82(3): 190–198.

32. Boulet, A. M. and Capecchi, M. R., Duplication of the Hoxd11 gene causes alterations in the axial and appendicular skeleton of the mouse. *Dev Biol*, 2002. 249(1): 96–107.

33. Olvera, D., et al., Pamidronate administration during pregnancy and lactation induces temporal preservation of maternal bone mass in a mouse model of osteogenesis imperfecta. *J Bone Miner Res*, 2019. 34(11): 2061–2074.

34. Briggs, M. D., Bell, P. A. and Pirog, K. A., The utility of mouse models to provide information regarding the pathomolecular mechanisms in human genetic skeletal diseases: the emerging role of endoplasmic reticulum stress (review). *Int J Mol Med*, 2015. 35(6): 1483–1492.

35. Bethune, M., Literature review and suggested protocol for managing ultrasound soft markers for Down syndrome: thickened nuchal fold, echogenic bowel, shortened femur, shortened humerus, pyelectasis and absent or hypoplastic nasal bone. *Australas Radiol*, 2007. 51(3): 218–225.

36. Rotten, D. and Levaillant, J. M., Two- and three-dimensional sonographic assessment of the fetal face. 2. *Analysis of cleft lip, alveolus and palate. Ultrasound Obstet Gynecol*, 2004. 24(4): 402–411.

37. Pilu, G., et al., Three-dimensional sonography of unilateral Tessier number 7 cleft in a mid-trimester fetus. *Ultrasound Obstet Gynecol*, 2005. 26(1): 98–99.

38. Buser, M. C. and Pohl, H. R., Windows of sensitivity to toxic chemicals in the development of cleft palates. *J Toxicol Environ Health B Crit Rev*, 2015. 18(5): 242–257.

39. Gritli-Linde, A., The etiopathogenesis of cleft lip and cleft palate: usefulness and caveats of mouse models. *Curr Top Dev Biol*, 2008. 84: 37–138.

40. Juriloff, D. M. and Harris, M. J., Mouse genetic models of cleft lip with or without cleft palate. *Birth Defects Res A Clin Mol Teratol*, 2008. 82(2): 63–77.

41. Pilu, G., et al., Diagnosis of midline anomalies of the fetal brain with the three-dimensional median view. *Ultrasound Obstet Gynecol*, 2006. 27(5): 522–529.

42. Boyd, P. A., et al., Evaluation of the prenatal diagnosis of neural tube defects by fetal ultrasonographic examination in different centres across Europe. *J Med Screen*, 2000. 7(4): 169–174.

43. Munoz, J. L., et al., Antenatal ultrasound compared to MRI evaluation of fetal myelomeningocele: a prenatal and postnatal evaluation. *J Perinat Med*, 2019. 47(7): 771–774.

44. Rigaud, M., et al., Species and strain differences in rodent sciatic nerve anatomy: implications for studies of neuropathic pain. *Pain*, 2008. 136(1–2): 188–201.

45. Hostikka, S. L., Gong, J. and Carpenter, E. M., Axial and appendicular skeletal transformations, ligament alterations, and motor neuron loss in Hoxc10 mutants. *Int J Biol Sci*, 2009. 5(5): 397–410.

46. Rolo, A., et al., Novel mouse model of encephalocele: post-neurulation origin and relationship to open neural tube defects. *Dis Model Mech*, 2019. 12(11).

47. Elbabaa, S. K., et al., First 60 fetal in-utero myelomeningocele repairs at Saint Louis Fetal Care Institute in the post-MOMS trial era: hydrocephalus treatment outcomes (endoscopic third ventriculostomy versus ventriculo-peritoneal shunt). *Childs Nerv Syst*, 2017. 33(7): 1157–1168.

48. Li, Z., et al., Morphologic evolution and coordinated development of the fetal lateral ventricles in the second and third trimesters. *AJNR Am J Neuroradiol*, 2019. 40(4): 718–725.

49. Wheway, G., et al., Aberrant Wnt signalling and cellular over-proliferation in a novel mouse model of Meckel-Gruber syndrome. *Dev Biol*, 2013. 377(1): 55–66.

50. Goulding, D. S., et al., Neonatal hydrocephalus leads to white matter neuroinflammation and injury in the corpus callosum of Ccdc39 hydrocephalic mice. *J Neurosurg Pediatr*, 2020, 25: 1–8.

6 Placenta Throughout Gestation

PLACENTA

Although the placenta is a temporary organ in an organism's life, it is a critical interface between the mother and fetus, providing gas exchange, nutrients, and serving as a barrier between the mother and fetus. As such, placental anomalies have often been associated with poor fetal health. Two of the most prevalent and morbid complications of human pregnancy -pre-eclampsia and fetal growth restriction -are associated with placental pathology.

The mouse is a reliable translational model to exam human placental disease, as the human and mouse placenta have several structural similarities (1). Primates and rodents have discoid or bi-discoid placenta, which is characterized by a single (discoid) disc (2). In both human and mouse pregnancies, the uterine arteries supply to maternal blood to the fetus. These arteries enter the placenta via larger spiral arteries, which then percolates through smaller capillary vasculature lined by fetal trophoblast; in this space, the feto-maternal exchange occurs. Humans and mice have a hemochorial placental type, which is the most invasive, with direct connection between the chorion and maternal blood. Mice and humans also have a hemochorial placenta, in which maternal blood comes in direct contact with trophoblast cells. Human placenta is hemomonochorial (one trophoblastic layer), while mouse placenta is hemotrichorial (three trophoblastic layers) (3). The umbilical vessels then connect the fetal capillaries to the fetus' main circulation (4).

HUMAN

In the human, a definitive placenta is only well visualized after 10–12 weeks gestation, as indicated by a focal thickening of hyperechoic tissue adjacent to the gestational sac (5). The chorion normally apposes with the amnion from 12 to 16 weeks.

Reference ranges for placental length and thickness during the second trimester have been shown to increase early detection of pregnancies which may results in intrauterine growth restriction or small for gestational age neonate (6). Factors such as uterine artery pulsatility index in the second trimester alone also help predict small for gestational age and possibility the risk of intrauterine fetal demise, or stillbirth (7,8). First trimester ultrasound has been shown to detect abnormally invasive placentation, when studied between 11 and 14 weeks gestation (9).

MOUSE

The mouse placenta is comprised of trophoblast cells and blood vessels; as in humans, the trophoblast cells develop from the outer layer of the embryo (trophectoderm). In mice, the chorioallantoic attachment occurs at 8.5 dpc, followed by the development and growth of the vascular network. This is the site of maternal fetal exchange that is equivalent to the human placenta villi (2,10). At 9.5 dpc, the chorio-allontoic fusion is completed, allowing for placental formation, and remodeling of the umbilical vessels to form the vein and artery. The mouse placenta gains full function capacity at around 10.5 dpc; at this time it is composed of three areas – the maternal decidua, the junctional zone and the labyrinth (11). The placenta has two vascular systems, maternal and fetal, and the appropriate perfusion is essential for exchanging of functions between them.

In the mouse, there are initially three vessels (one artery and two veins) in the vitelline portion of the umbilical cord, which is closest to the placenta. However, at the fetal or allantoic portion, the umbilical cord contains one artery and one vein. Thus, most color Doppler of the umbilical cord in the mouse fetus has two vessels. The umbilical artery and the umbilical vein form at 9.5 dpc and are subsequently easy to identify on ultrasound.

PLACENTAL ANOMALIES

A range of placental anomalies detected via ultrasonography have been directly linked to poor maternal and/or fetal outcomes.

Placenta Accreta/Percreta/Increta

As cesarean rates have increased, the incidence of abnormal placentation has been rising (12). Placenta accreta can be detected as early as 15–20 weeks of gestation, usually by visualizing placental lacunae, which are vascular spaces within the placenta (13).

Placental Calcifications

As the placenta matures, small calcifications, which appear as small bright echogenic areas in the placenta can be visualized. Premature or accelerated placental calcifications have been associated with pre-eclampsia, maternal hypertension, and intra uterine growth restriction.

Cord Insertion

The umbilical cord normally inserts into the central portion of the placenta, away from the placental edge. Abnormalities in the umbilical cord entry can includes marginal umbilical cord entry abnormity or velamentous umbilical cord entry abnormity, in which umbilical vessels diverge as they traverse between the amnion and chorion before reaching the placenta. In humans, color Doppler has been a very useful tool to evaluate and diagnose these conditions (14). Some cord anomalies have been associated with fetal growth restriction and preterm labor (15). See further Figs. 6.1–6.22.

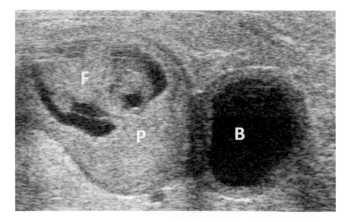

FIGURE 6.1 At 9.5 dpc, the mouse placenta is finally developed enough to appreciate via ultrasonography. The placental location (P) can be determined by visualization of a thickened of one part of the myometrium . Additionally, the gestational sac appears to have a "straighter" and less-rounded edge at the location of the developing placenta. At this early gestational age the only characteristic of the placenta that can be detected by ultrasound is the location. The maternal bladder (B) is also shown in this view for comparison. The umbilical artery and the umbilical vein form at 9.5 dpc and are subsequently easy to identify on ultrasound as a linear structure traversing from the embryo to the sidewall of the uterus, inserting into the developing placenta.

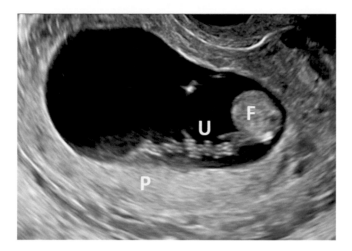

FIGURE 6.2 In the human, the earliest that the human placental location can be determined is at 8–9 weeks gestation. The placental location (P) can be noted by both the location of the umbilical cord (U) traversing from the fetus (F) to its insertion into the uterine wall. These characteristics correlate to mouse imaging at this stage, in which the thickened of one part of the myometrium indicates the placental location.

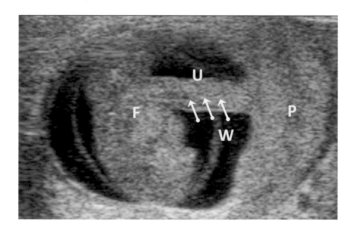

FIGURE 6.3 In the mouse on 10.5 dpc, the umbilical cord (U) is reliably visualized and provides additional confirmation of the placental location (P). The two vessels (the umbilical artery and vein) are able to be indentified, with the vessel walls (W) appearing as a hyperechoic line providing a visual separation of these two vessels. At this gestational age, the site and location of the umbilical cord insertion (I) into the placenta can begin to be assessed for appropriate central placement.

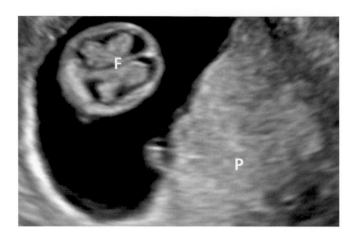

FIGURE 6.4 In the human at 12 weeks, the placenta (P) becomes more distinguishable, as a slightly more hyperechoic and discoid shape, which creates a "flattened" surface of the uterine wall. The development and sonographic findings of the human placenta at this stage are very similar to that of the mouse placenta. The fetal head (F) and brain can be seen, for comparison.

(a)   (b)

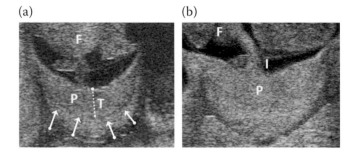

FIGURE 6.5 **A:** By 11.5 dpc in the mouse, the fetus (F) as well as the margins of the placenta (P) are visible, as shown at the tips of the white arrows. Even at this early gestational age, it is possible to determine the placental thickness, as shown here (T). **B:** Placental thickness is measured perpendicular to the uterine wall and through the placenta at the site of umbilical cord insertion (I).

(a)   (b)

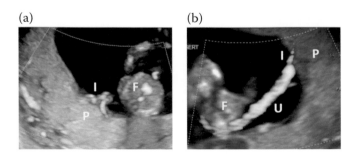

FIGURE 6.6 **AB:** In the early second trimester in the human, the umbilical cord insertion site (I) into the placenta as well as the umbilical cord (U) blood flow are easily detected. This allows for the location of the umbilical cord from the fetus (F) to the placental insertion site (P) to be determined.

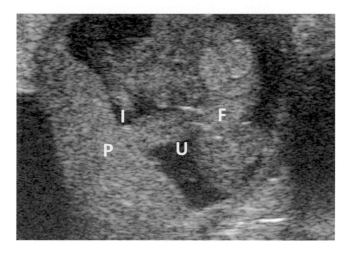

FIGURE 6.7 At 12.5 dpc in the mouse, the placenta continues its growth and establishment. The umbilical cord insertion (I) into the appropriate location at the center of the placenta confirms the normal insertion of the umbilical cord. Even as the fetus (F) continues its rapid development, the umbilical cord (U) traversing from the fetus to the placenta (P) continues to be visualized with ease.

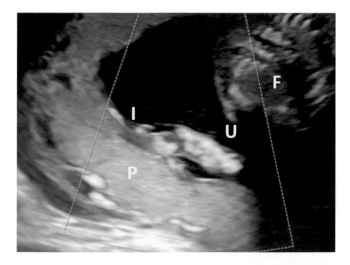

FIGURE 6.8 At 18 weeks gestation in the human, the umbilical cord insertion into the abdomen is visible. The umbilical cord insertion into the center of the placenta can still be easily seen into the center of the placenta, demonstrating normal insertion of the umbilical cord. Even at the fetus (F) continues its rapid development, the umbilical cord (U) traversing from the fetus to the placenta (P) continues to be visualized.

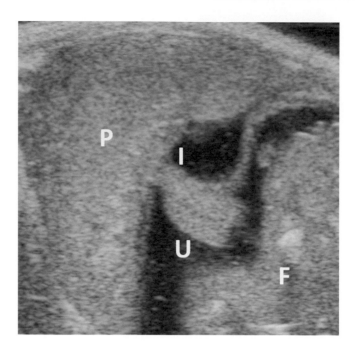

FIGURE 6.9   By 13.5 dpc in the mouse, both the placenta and the fetus (F) have continued to rapidly grow in size. The placental location (P) is easily seen in the sagittal view, as a discoid shape. The umbilical cord (U) and insertion site (I) into the placenta is less reliably seen at this gestational age, due to the decreased free space within the amniotic sac.

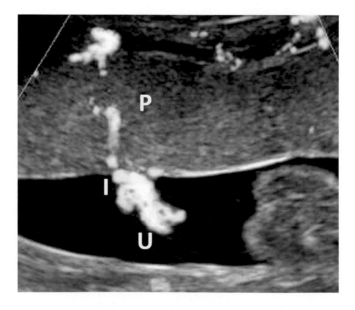

FIGURE 6.10   In the human around 20 weeks gestation, the placenta has grown in size and the placental shape begins to appear more well-defined. The placental location (P) is easily seen in the sagittal view, as a discoid shape, much thicker than the neighboring myometrial wall, and with the umbilical cord (U) and its insertion site (I) still easily visible with color Doppler flow.

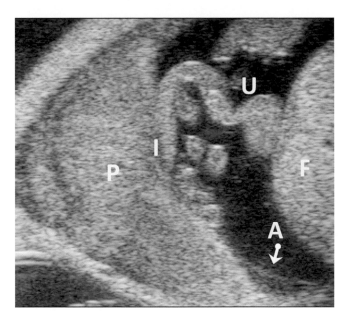

FIGURE 6.11   At 14.5 dpc in the mouse the umbilical cord attachment is clearly seen from the fetal abdomen (F) with the umbilical cord insertion site into the placenta (I) located in the expected position in the middle or central portion of the placenta (P). The amniotic membrane (A) still visible, yet to fuse with the myometrial wall at this gestational stage. At this gestational age, the umbilical cord has become longer, more coiled and tortuous in appearance; the two vessels of the umbilical cord can be distinguished in some views. The umbilical cord can be seen here traversing from the fetus to placental insertion in a cork-screw fashion.

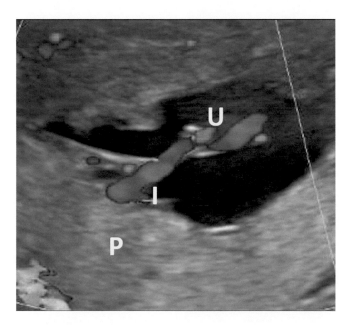

FIGURE 6.12   Human mid gestation 28 weeks and 2 days and marginal cord insertion; umbilical cord insertion site into the placenta (I) is not located on the central portion, but is considered a marginal cord insertion, as it is not located in the expected position in the middle or central portion of the placenta (P). At this gestational age, similar to the mouse, the umbilical cord has elongated into its distinct coiled and tortuous appearance. The umbilical cord can be seen here traversing from the fetus to placental insertion in a cork-screw fashion. Similar to the mouse, the placenta at this gestational age is homogenous. Both the mouse and the human placenta in these images represent a posterior placenta location.

(a)   (b)

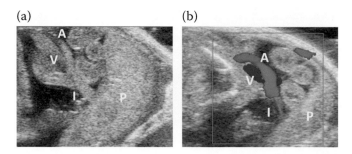

FIGURE 6.13 AB: In the mouse at 15.5 dpc, the edges of the placenta are easily demarcated; measurements such as the mid placenta thickness (T) can still be easily obtained in a sagittal section. The planes of the placenta are also readily determined. Due to the rapid growth of the fetus, the fetus and placenta are usually abutting. In the mouse at 15.5 dpc, the two vessels of the umbilical cord – artery (A) and vein (V) – are seen coiled in the basic gray-scale ultrasound (left), coarsing from the fetal side (F) to the placenta (P). Application of color doppler permits detection of the arterial and venous flow in each vessel, offering further clarity of the location and relationship of the vessels from the fetal abdomen to their insertion into the placenta. Of note, humans have three vessels in the umbilical cord, having two arteries and one vein; the mouse has two vessels.

(a)   (b)

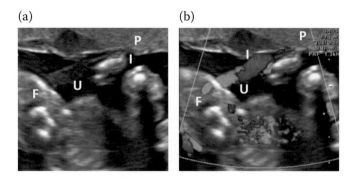

FIGURE 6.14 A: In the human during the second trimester, the basic gray-scale ultrasound allows for indentification of the placental location, size and planes (P). **B:** Application of color doppler permits detection of the blood flow, offering further clarity of the location and relationship of the insertion of the umbilical cord vessels into their insertion (I) into the placenta (P).

(a)   (b)

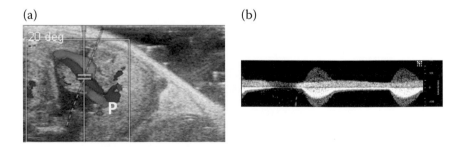

FIGURE 6.15 AB: In the mouse at 15.5 dpc, the two umbilical vessels are seen with Doppler cord pulses, showing the two vessels entwined. In A, addition of the color Doppler allows for discrete identification of the umbilical artery and vein as they coil around each other and traverse from the fetus to the umbilical cord. In B, the Doppler transducer and beam angle are shown, applied to the pulsating vessel of interest (in the example above, the umbilical artery).

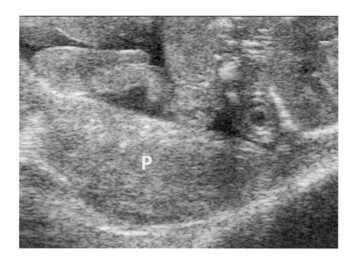

FIGURE 6.16 In the mouse at 16.5 dpc, the size, borders and location of the placenta (P) are still easily demarcated; in this representation, the placenta is shown to be in a posterior placenta location. As the ultrasound is placed on the anterior or ventral portion of the maternal abdomen, the images at the top of the frame are closest to the ultrasound probe, and thus the most anterior. Consequently, the images that are at the bottom of the image from are that are farthest from the beam, and as such, correlate to the a more posterior location within the abdomen. In this example, the placenta is at the bottom of the frame, and thus is considered a posterior placental location.

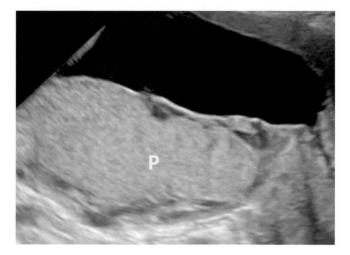

FIGURE 6.17 In this late third-trimester image in the human, the placenta (P) is noted to be at the bottom of the frame, and thus in a posterior location within the uterus. This represents a posterior placenta, very similar to the mouse ultrasound as shown above. Again, the size, borders and location of the placenta (P) are still easily demarcated at this gestational age.

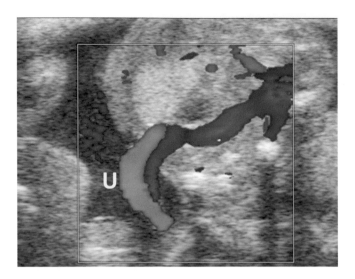

FIGURE 6.18   In the mouse at 16.5 dpc, the color Doppler ultrasound shows the coiled, two vessel umbilical cord (U) as it inserts into the fetal abdomen. The color Doppler allows for distinct umbilical cord flow into the large fetal internal blood vessels. The insertion of the cord into the fetal abdomen and entrance into the fetal vascular circulation is seen.

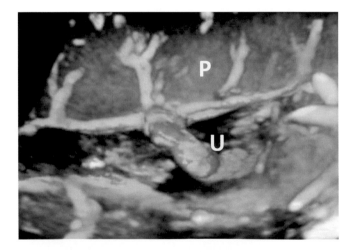

FIGURE 6.19   The human placenta during the third trimester has a strong establishment of the placental blood vessels, seen as the umbilical cord (U) and placental vessels connect, which lead into the maternal/fetal barrier. One umbilical vein carries oxygenated blood from the placenta (P) to the fetus, while two umbilical arteries carry deoxygenated blood from the fetus to the placenta. The vessels at the top of the image are shown diving into the intervillous space.

(a) (b)

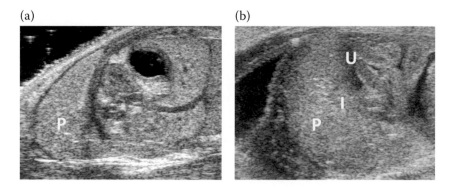

FIGURE 6.20 AB: In the mouse at 17.5 dpc, the placenta (P) begins to become more heterogenic – with smaller punctate echogenic areas seen – and less homogenous at this stage. The size and location of placenta is still well demarcated, in addition to the insertion (I) of the umbilical cord into the central region of the placenta. The wall and lumen of the umbilical cord (U) are both easily identified.

(a) (b)

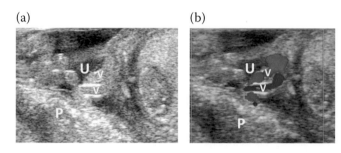

FIGURE 6.21 In the mouse at 18.5 dpc, the placenta (P) and umbilical cord (U) are still able to be identified. Application of color Doppler demonstrates the fetal cord insertion of the artery and vein into the fetus. (A) The two vessels (V) of umbilical cord can be seen in the grays-cale but are more easily distinguished when color Doppler is applied (B).

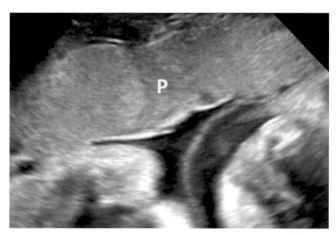

FIGURE 6.22 In the human late third trimester (shown here at 35 weeks gestation), the placenta (P) is seen here in an anterior location (i.e., located on the anterior wall). Similar to the mouse at this late gestational age, the fetal structures, umbilical cord and placenta are all in close proximity, as the structure are more compressed together. Consequently, measurements of the placental size and location, as well as the umbilical cord insertion become more challenging to obtain.

REFERENCES

1. Cox, B., Kotlyar, M., Evangelou, A. I., Ignatchenko, V., Ignatchenko, A., Whiteley, K., et al., Comparative systems biology of human and mouse as a tool to guide the modeling of human placental pathology. *Mol Syst Biol.* 2009. 5: 279.

2. Soncin, F., Natale, D. and Parast, M.M., Signaling pathways in mouse and human trophoblast differentiation: a comparative review. *Cell Mol Life Sci.* 2015. 72(7): 1291–1302.

3. Furukawa, S., Kuroda, Y. and Sugiyama, A., A comparison of the histological structure of the placenta in experimental animals. *J Toxicol Pathol.* 2014. 27(1): 11–18.

4. Georgiades, P., Ferguson-Smith, A. C. and Burton, G.J., Comparative developmental anatomy of the murine and human definitive placentae. *Placenta.* 2002. 23(1): 3–19.

5. Kurjak, A. and Kupesic, S. Doppler assessment of the intervillous blood flow in normal and abnormal early pregnancy. *Obstet Gynecol.* 1997. 89(2): 252–256.

6. McGinty, P., Farah, N., Dwyer, V. O., Hogan, J., Reilly, A., Turner, M.J., et al., Ultrasound assessment of placental function: the effectiveness of placental biometry in a low-risk population as a predictor of a small for gestational age neonate. *Prenat Diagn.* 2012. 32(7): 620–626.

7. Allen, R. E., Morlando, M., Thilaganathan, B., Zamora, J., Khan, K. S., Thangaratinam, S., et al., Predictive accuracy of second-trimester uterine artery Doppler indices for stillbirth: a systematic review and meta-analysis. *Ultrasound Obstet Gynecol.* 2016. 47(1): 22–27.

8. Familiari, A., Bhide, A., Morlando, M., Scala, C., Khalil, A. and Thilaganathan, B., Mid-pregnancy fetal biometry, uterine artery Doppler indices and maternal demographic characteristics: role in prediction of small-for-gestational-age birth. *Acta Obstet Gynecol Scand.* 2016. 95(2): 238–244.

9. Cali, G., Forlani, F., Foti, F., Minneci, G., Manzoli, L., Flacco, M. E., et al., Diagnostic accuracy of first-trimester ultrasound in detecting abnormally invasive placenta in high-risk women with placenta previa. *Ultrasound Obstet Gynecol.* 2018. 52(2): 258–264.

10. Watson, E. D. and Cross, J. C., Development of structures and transport functions in the mouse placenta. *Physiology (Bethesda).* 2005. 20: 180–193.

11. Adamson, S. L., Lu, Y., Whiteley, K. J., Holmyard, D., Hemberger, M., Pfarrer, C., et al., Interactions between trophoblast cells and the maternal and fetal circulation in the mouse placenta. *Dev Biol.* 2002. 250(2): 358–373.

12. Papanikolaou, I. G., Domali, E., Daskalakis, G., Theodora, M., Telaki, E., Drakakis, P., et al., Abnormal placentation: current evidence and review of the literature. *Eur J Obstet Gynecol Reprod Biol.* 2018. 228: 98–105.

13. Comstock, C. H., Love, J. J. Jr., Bronsteen, R. A., Lee, W., Vettraino, I. M., Huang, R. R., et al., Sonographic detection of placenta accreta in the second and third trimesters of pregnancy. *Am J Obstet Gynecol.* 2004. 190(4): 1135–1140.

14. Sun, J., Wang, L. and Li, Y., Clinical value of color doppler ultrasound in prenatal diagnosis of umbilical cord entry abnormity. *Pak J Med Sci.* 2016. 32(6): 1414–1418.

15. Hasegawa, J., Matsuoka, R., Ichizuka, K., Sekizawa, A. and Okai, T., Ultrasound diagnosis and management of umbilical cord abnormalities. *Taiwan J Obstet Gynecol.* 2009. 48(1): 23–27.

Index

A

achondroplasia, 18
anembryonic pregnancy (blighted ovum), 9
average mean diameter, myometrium, 12*f*

B

bone malformations, 18
bone morphogenetic proteins (BMP), 37
brain: anomalies, 55–57;
    human, 52–53;
    mouse, 53–54;
    views of, mouse and human, 52*f*–57*f*
brain/CNS: anomalies, 70;
    human, 69–70;
    mouse, 70;
    views of, 69*f*–71*f*;

C

cardiac: four chambers of heart, 32*f*
    human, 31;
    humans and mice, 31–33;
    mouse heart tube formation, 32
cardiac activity, establish, detection and quantification of:
        human, 7
    human, 8*f*;
    mouse, 7;
    views of, 7*f*–8*f*
central nervous system and facial development:
        anomalies, 50;
    brain, 52–57;
    central nervous system and facial development, 45;
    eye, human and mouse, 46*f*–48, 49*f*;
    imaging of central nervous system (CNS) and facial
        development, 45;
    mouse, 50;
    nasal structures and palate, 45;
    spine, 48;
craniofacial anomalies, 25–26;
    views of, 25*f*–26*lf*
CRL (crown to rump length): human 11 weeks, 23*f*;
    human 12 weeks gestation, 23*f*;
    human normal and abnormal pregnancies, 23*f*;
    mouse 11.5 dpc, 23*f*;
    mouse 12.5 dpc, 23*f*
crown rump length (CRL), 5–7, *See* CRL (crown to rump
    length)

D

Dandy-Walker malformation, 70;

decidualization and early implantation, 2–4;
    gestational sac, development of, 4–5;
    human, 2;
    mouse, 2;
    views of, 3–4*f*
dichorionic twins, 26;

E

early murine fetal growth curve, 10–12;
early pregnancy loss, 9;
    failed pregnancies 8.5 to 13.5 dpc, 11*f*
endrometrium, 2–4
extremities: human long bones, 36;
    mouse humerus, 37;
    paw and hand anomalies, 37
eye: anomalies, 48;
    facial development, human and mouse, 46*f*–48*f*;
    human, 47;
    mouse, 48
eye, human and mouse, views of, 46*f*–47*f*, 49*f*
eye and orbit: anomalies, 63;
    human, 61–62;
    mouse, 62;
    views of, 61*f*–63*f*

F

face and snout: human, 66–67;
    mouse, 67–68;
    views of, 67*f*
failed pregnancies, views of, 11*f*
fetal demise, normal and abnormal fetal growth: first
        trimester fetal growth anomalies, 21;
    human pregnancy CLR 10 weeks gestation, 22*f*;
    mouse, 22, 22*f*;
    mouse forelimb paw hands with digits 11.5 dpc, 21*f*;
    – put this with limbs, hands paws listing
    human, 19–21
fetal growth anomalies, first trimester, 21–25
fetal heart rate, 8–9;
    views of, 9*f*
fetal polarity and development: human, 7;
    mouse, 7
fetal pole, detection of, 5;
    human, 6;
    mouse, 6;
    views of, 6*f*
first trimester complications: anembryonic pregnancy
        (blighted ovum), 9–10
    early pregnancy loss, 9;
    first trimester spontaneous abortion, 10

G

gestational sac, mouse, 4–5
gestational sac, development of, 1;
    defined, 4;
    human, 4;
    mouse, 4–5;
    views of, 4f–5f

H

head and face, 21–25;
    human, 21–22;
    views of, 22f–24f
heart: anomalies, 61;
    human, 60–61;
    mouse, 61
human: 28 weeks and 2 days, marginal cord insertion, 81f;
    abnormal pregnancy 8 weeks 5 days, 24f;
    anembryonic pregnancy weeks 1 day, 10f;
    arm, radius (R) and ulna (U) 12 weeks, 20f;
    arterial and venous flow patters, umbilical cord, 17f;
    both shoulders and upper limbs 11-12 weeks, 20f;
    brain stem and spine mid gestational age, 50f;
    cardiac anatomy 10 to 11 weeks, 16f;
    cartilage, end of bones in hands second trimester, 39f;
    cerebullum (CB), falx cerebri (Falx), posterior horn of the lateral ventricle (LV), 55f;
    CRL 11 weeks, 23f;
    CRL sagittal or "profile view", 23f;
    crown (C) and rump (R) CRL 10 weeks, 22f;
    diaphragm, dividing heart (H) and intestines, 36f;
    diaphragm 13.5 dpc, 35f;
    discrete ventricular structure 10 to 11 weeks, 16f;
    eye anatomy midgestation, 49f;
    fetal cardiac activity 6 weeks 1 day, 9f;
    fetal foot 18 weeks gestation, 40f;
    fetal heart, 62f;
    fetal pole 6 weeks 3 days, 6f;
    first limb buds 8-10 weeks, 19f;
    foot, 40f;
    fourth ventricle (FV), third ventricle (TV), thalamus (TH), midline falx cerebri (Falx) and laterventricle (LV) 14.5 dpc, 55f;
    hands second trimester, 38f;
    human endometrium, 3f;
    human placental location 8-9 weeks gestation, 77f;
    identification of spinal anomalies or neural tube defects, 52f;
    lens of the eye (L), bones of the orbit, nasal bones, 64f;
    midgestational brain antomy, 56f;
    mid gestation humerus (H), 42f;
    midgestation posterior brain structures, 57f;
    midline vertebral and lateral vertebral arches, 51f;
    nasal bridge (N), maxilla (MX), and mandible 11 weeks, 26f;
    non-pregnant uterus, human and mouse, 2f;
    placenta (P) in anterior location 35 weeks gestation, 85f;
    placenta 12 weeks, 78f;
    placenta growth 20 weeks, 80f;
    placental blood vessels third trimester, 84f;
    placental location, size and plane second trimester, 82f;
    pregnancy 8 weeks 2 days, 8f;
    pregnancy 8 weeks 6 days, 24f;
    pregnancy CRL 11.5 weeks, 22f;
    prenancy dichorionic diamniotic (di/di) 12 weeks, 27f;
    profile 10-11 weeks, 25f;
    profile 14 weeks, 32f, 46f;
    profile image forth ventricle (FV), cerebellum (CB), medulla oblongata (MO) early second trimester, 53f;
    right and left ventricles, 33f;
    sagittal plane view of face 4 weeks, 46f–47f;
    sagittal view, 33f;
    second trimesters, ventricles, 34f;
    third-trimester placenta (P), 83f;
    tibia (Tib), fibula (Fib) and femur, 41f;
    transaxial plane view of face, BOD measurements, 49f;
    transverse axial plane view of brain second trimester, 54f;
    twins 10 weeks, 27f;
    umbilical cord (U), 78f;
    umbilical cord insertion 18 weeks, 79f;
    upper extremity long bones, 43f

I

Imaging techniques, 1
implantation and embryonic imaging: dating, mouse and human, 1;
    decidualization and early implantation, 2–5;
    detection of a fetal pole, 5–6;
    development of gestational sac, 4–5;
    fetal heart rate, 8–9;
    fetal polarity and development, 7–8;
    imaging, 1;
    preimplantation development, 1;
    views of, 8f–9f
implantation and imagining, mouse 4.5-9.5 dpc, humans 5-9 weeks, fetal heart rate, 8

K

kidneys: anomalies, 59;
    human, 59;
    mouse, 59;
    views of, 59f–60f

L

lamba sign, 26
late-gestation and third trimester: eye and orbit, 61–63;
    face and snout, 66–68;
    heart, 60–61;
    kidneys, 59–60;
    limbs, hands, feet and paws, 63–66
limb buds: human, 16–18;
    mouse forelimbs and hind limb buds, 18;
    views of, 17f–19f
limbs, hands, feet and paws: anomalies, 65;
    human, 64;
    mouse, 64;
    overview, 63–64;
    views of, 64f–66f
limbs development, views of, 19f–21f

M

mean sac diameter (MSD), 4
median nasal process (MNP), 22
mega cisterna magna, 70
mid-gestation and second trimester: cardiac
        anomalies, 33–34;
    diaphragm, 34–36;
    extremities, 36–43;
    imaging, 31;
    limb and digits growth and anomalies, human and
        mouse, 37f–43f;
    long bone and limb anomalies, 37–43;
    organogenesis, 31
missing limbs, 18
monozygotic twinning, 28
mouse: (multiple pregnancy) gestational sac 9.5 dpc, 27f;
    abnormal pregnancy CRL 12.5 dpc, 24f;
    anembryonic pregnancy 8.5 dpc, 10f;
    brain anatomy 15.5 dpc, 56f;
    brain structures 17.5 dpc, 70f;
    cardiac anatomy 18.5 dpc, 63f;
    caudal region with vertebral processes, 51f;
    centra, 65f;
    coronal plane 15.5 dpc, 48f;
    CRL 11.5 dpc, 23f;
    CRL 12.5 dpc, 24f;
    crown (C and rump (R) CRL 10.5 dpc, 22f;
    diaphragm 13.5 dpc, 35f;
    edges of placenta 15.5 days, 82f;
    elongated humerus 14.5 dpc, 41f;
    eye anatomy 15.5 dpc, 49f;
    failed pregnancies 8.5 to 13.5 dpc, 11f;
    femurs, 66f;
    fetal cardiac activity 9.5 dpc, 9f;
    fetal heart 16.5 dpc, 62f;
    fetal pole, gestational sac 8.5 dpc, 6f;
    fetus 9.5 dpc, 8f;
    first detection of limb buds 10.5 dpc, 19f;
    forelimb buds 11.5 dpc, 20f;
    forelimb paw hands 12.5 dpc, 21f;
    four chambers of the heart 13.5 dpc, 32f;
    growth of cardiac structures 15.5 dpc, 34f;
    heart (H) above diaphragm 15.5 dpc, 36f;
    heart, ventricular septum (S) 14.5 dpc, 33f;
    hind limb paw 13.5 dpc, 39f;
    humerus (H) 17.5 dpc, 66f;
    interdigitary apoptosis paw hands, 38f;
    intervening uterus 11.5 dpc, 28f;
    lateral ventricle (LV) and fourth ventricle (FV),
        mesencephalic ventricle (MV and third ventricle
        ((TV) 13.5 doc, 52f;
    lens of the eye (L), bones of the orbit,nasal bones (N)
        17.5 dpc, 64f;
    mandible, maxilla and median nasal process (MNP)
        12.5 dpc, 26f;
    mouse fetal bladder, 60f;
    mouse fetal tail, 70f;
    paw digits (D), 65f;
    paw hands 13.5 dpc, 37f;
    placenta (P) and umbilical cord (U), 85f;
    placenta, size and location 17.5 dpc, 85f;
    placenta 9.5 dpc, 76f;

    placenta 12.5 dpc, 79f;
    placenta and fetus (F) 13.5 dpc, 80f;
    placental margins 11.5 dpc, 78f;
    posterior fossa (PF), cervical (Cv), thoracic (T) and
        sacral (S) spine, 69f;
    pregnancy 3.5 dpc, 3f;
    pregnancy 4.5 dpc, 3f;
    pregnancy 5.5 dpc, 4f;
    pregnancy 6.5 dpc, 4f;
    profile 10.5 dpc, 25f;
    profile 13.5 dpc, 46f;
    right ulna (U) and radius bones (R) 16.5 dpc, 66f;
    sagittal image of third ventricle (TV), mesencephalic
        ventricle (MV), pons (PO) and medulla
        oblongata 14.5 dpc, 54f;
    sagittal plane (left), fetal snout 16.5, 68f;
    sagittal plane view of face 13.5 dpc, 46f–47f;
    sagittal view with posterior fossa and spinal cord 13.5
        dpc, 50f;
    size, borders and location of placenta, 83f;
    spine (Spine) flanked by two kidneys 16.5 dpc, 60f;
    spine 15.5 dpc, 51f;
    tibia (T) and fibula (Fib), 66f;
    tibia (T), fibia (F) and femur can be measured 14.5
        dpc, 41f;
    transaxial plane view of face, BOD measurements 14.5
        dpc, 49f;
    transverse image of brain, 53f;
    two chamber of the heart 11.5 dpc, 17f;
    two vessel umbilical cords 12.5 dpc, 18f;
    two vessel umbilical cords 16.5 dpc, 84f;
    ulna of the upper limb 15.5 dpc, 42f;
    umbilical cord (U), 77f;
    umbilical cord attachment 14.5 dpc, 81f;
    ventricles of the heart, 61f;
    vitreous humor (V), retina (R), and lens (L) 18.5
        dpc, 64f
mouse CRL 12.5 dpc, 24f
multifetal gestation and pregnancy spacing: 12 weeks
        gestation di-di pregnancy, 27f;
    human, 26–27;
    human twin gestation 10 weeks, di-di pregancy, 27f;
    mouse, 28, 28f;
    mouse 9.5 dpc separation of gestational sac, 27f;
    mouse pregnancy 11.5 dpc, intervening uterus, 28f;
    views of, 26f–28f
murine fetal development curve, 12f
myometrium, 12f

N

nasal structures and palate: anomalies, 46;
    human palate, 45–46;
    mouse secondary palate, 46
neural tube defects (NTDs), 50

O

organogenesis, 7
    – put this under placenta
    mouse two vessel umbilical cord 12.5 dpc, 18f
organogenesis, first trimester: cardiac, 15;
    cardiac anomalies, 16;

human, 15;
imaging, 15;
limb buds, 16;
mouse, 16;
organogenesis, 15;
vies of, 16*f*;
views of, 17*f*
organogenesis and first trimester: fetal demise, normal and
        abnormal fetal growth, 18–21;
    head and face, 21–25;

P

placenta, 75
placenta accreta/percreta/increta, 76
placenta throughout gestation: cord insertion, 76;
    human, 75;
    mouse, 75–76;
    placenta, 75;
    placenta accreta/percreta/increta, 76;
    placental anomalies, 76;
    placental calcifications, 76;
    views of, 76*f*–85*f*
placenta types, 26

posterior fossa pathologies, 70
preimplantation development, views of, 2*f*
primordial heart, 7
    – move to "cardiac"

S

skeletal dysplasias, 18
spina bifida, 50
spine: human, 49
    views of, 50*f*–52*f*;
spine and tail: anomalies, 69;
    human, 68;
    mouse, 69;
    views of, 68*f*
spontaneous abortion, first trimester, 10

T

T-sign, 26

Y

yolk sac, 5*f*